Writing Nursing Diagnoses

A Critical Thinking Approach

Writing Nursing Diagnoses

A Critical Thinking Approach

Idolia Cox Collier, DNSc, RNCS
Associate Professor
University of New Mexico
College of Nursing
Albuquerque, New Mexico

Katheryn E. McCash, RNC, MSN
Instructor
University of New Mexico
College of Nursing
Albuquerque, New Mexico

Joanne Marino Bartram, RN, MS
Instructor
University of New Mexico
College of Nursing
Albuquerque, New Mexico

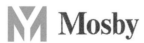 Mosby

St. Louis   Baltimore   Boston   Carlsbad   Chicago   Naples   New York   Philadelphia   Portland
London   Madrid   Mexico City   Singapore   Sydney   Tokyo   Toronto   Wiesbaden

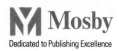

Mosby
Dedicated to Publishing Excellence

A Times Mirror
Company

Publisher: Nancy L. Coon
Editor: Loren Wilson
Project Manager: Dana Peick
Production Editor: Stavra Demetrulias
Designers: Liz Fett/Amy Buxton
Cover Designer: Amy Buxton

A NOTE TO THE READER:

The author and publisher have made every attempt to check dosages and nursing content for accuracy. Because the science of pharmacology is continually advancing, our knowledge base continues to expand. Therefore we recommend that the reader always check product information for changes in dosage or administration before administering any medication. This is particularly important with new or rarely used drugs.

Printed in the United States of America

Composition by Wm. C. Brown
Printing/binding by Western Publishing

Mosby-Year Book, Inc.
11830 Westline Industrial Drive
St. Louis, Missouri 63146

Library of Congress Cataloging-in-Publication Data

Collier, Idolia Cox.
    Writing nursing diagnoses : a critical thinking approach / Idolia
Cox Collier, Katheryn E. McCash, Joanne Marino Bartram. —1st ed.
        p.   cm.
    Includes bibliographical references and index.
    ISBN 0–8151–1639–X
    1. Nursing diagnosis.   2. Nursing—Authorship.   I. McCash,
Katheryn E.   II. Bartram, Joanne Marino.   III. Title.
    [DNLM: 1. Nursing Diagnosis—methods.   2. Writing.   3. Thinking.
WY 100.4 C699w 1996]
RT48.6.C65   1996
610.73—dc20
DNLM/DLC
for Library of Congress   95–46011
                                                                  CIP

Preface

Students need help in learning to write accurate nursing diagnoses. Like learning a second language, new cognitive skills and vocabulary need to be practiced again and again until proficiency is gained. *WRITING NURSING DIAGNOSES: A Critical Thinking Approach* was written to provide students with an organized and logical way to gain this proficiency.

Students and practicing nurses can use this book to practice writing nursing diagnoses. For the true beginner, the first sections of the text provide the necessary background needed to begin writing diagnoses. For the nurse with a basic knowledge of the principles of writing nursing diagnoses, the front sections provide a refresher of the theory base of nursing diagnosis. For all nurses from student and novice to expert clinician, the cases offer interesting and challenging ways to practice the critical thinking skills associated with writing accurate nursing diagnoses.

Many special features have been incorporated into the book to aid the learning process. These features include:

1. Case study approach: This approach to learning is a favorite of students because it removes learning from the realm of theory and makes it a practical and relevant technique by using situations that mimic clinical practice.

2. Interactional: Following presentation of the theoretical content in the first chapters of the book, all subsequent material is presented in an interactional format. The student is asked a series of questions and is expected to write directly in the casebook in the space provided. The user-friendly design is meant to invite interaction and make the learning experience a personal one.

3. Critical thinking challenges of increasing complexity: The learner is helped to use a critical thinking approach to writing accurate diagnoses by the nature of the questions in the cases. While most diagnoses are neither simple nor complex in and of themselves, the cases and subsequent critical thinking questions are leveled so the learner is brought steadily from the simple to the complex. Cases and questions are presented at three levels of complexity—simple, moderate, and complex. Once the learner completes a level, the associated cognitive skills are applied in the next level of cases. In this way, knowledge and skills accumulate over the course of the cases.

4. Focus on accuracy: The idea of accuracy of nursing diagnosis is presented initially in the front matter of the book. The work of Lunney is cited and used throughout the text as the reference point for accuracy. The emphasis on accuracy continues in every case when the student is challenged to write the most accurate diagnoses in a given case.

5. Detailed answers provided: Detailed and complete answers are provided to all questions asked of the learner. In this way, the student feels challenged to "beat the experts" while learning the process. It is expected that, as the learner becomes more accurate in responding to the questions, there will be less and less disparity in the responses of the learner and the experts. Concurrence of responses will provide positive feedback to the learner, while incongruity will add extra challenge and incentive.

6. NANDA-based nursing diagnoses: It was the decision of the authors to use the diagnoses, definitions, and defining characteristics of the North American Nursing Diagnosis Association (NANDA) as the "gold standard" for the cases. Although there are many excellent nursing diagnosis books available, use of the NANDA data base reduces confusion and promotes consistency. Where appropriate, other theoretical approaches are discussed.

The book is organized into Parts and Chapters. Part One consists of three chapters that focus on the theoretical foundation of writing accurate diagnoses. These early chapters discuss the nursing process, guidelines for writing nursing diagnoses, and the process of making an accurate nursing diagnosis. Part Two consists of three chapters that are aimed at assisting the student to get started writing nursing diagnoses, building confidence in that ability, and finally, gaining expertise in analyzing more complex cases.

We owe a special thanks to our editor, Loren Wilson, for her advice and assistance along the way. On the homefront, we must thank our families for their support and understanding. Our conscientious reviewers—Pauline Green, Tamara Rice, and Gayle Varnell—provided valuable insight and practical suggestions on both the case studies themselves and our interpretation of accurate nursing diagnoses. Our hardworking typists—Loretta Campbell and Connie Robb—earn special thanks and praise. We also owe each other a hearty pat on the back for the perseverance and determination that stayed with us from start to finish of this project.

Idolia Cox Collier
Katheryn E. McCash
Joanne Marino Bartram

Contents

Introduction

Nursing Process and Critical Thinking

Nursing Process

Nursing is a complex and challenging discipline. Professional nurses deal with more than just diseases and technology. They deal with the full range of human responses to actual or potential health problems.[1] This is a complex and broadly defined scope of practice. Nurses must use critical thinking skills to confront the wide variety of client issues, problems, and needs that arise in everyday nursing practice. The nursing process has evolved as a tool to assist nurses with professional practice. It is the framework within which nurses organize information about client problems and design interventions to meet client needs.

The **nursing process** is an assertive, problem-solving approach to the identification and treatment of client problems. It provides an organizing framework for the knowledge, thoughts, and actions that nurses bring to client care. Within this framework nurses apply their general clinical knowledge base to specific client situations. The result is comprehensive and individualized nursing care. Regardless of their area of clinical expertise, all nurses must become proficient in the use of the nursing process.

Components of the Nursing Process

The nursing process has five steps: assessment, diagnosis, planning, implementation, and evaluation. Each step requires the use of specialized nursing knowledge, critical thinking skills, a client-specific focus, creativity, flexibility, and caring. Examining each step individually is a logical way to learn about the nursing process but not a true reflection of the process in practice. In practice the steps are not always linear or discrete. In other words, they do not always occur in sequence, one step after the other. They may overlap or occur out of sequence. This is particularly true for the assessment step. This step may need to be repeated at several points throughout the process as the nurse identifies the need for additional data about the client. The evaluation step is another component of the nursing process that may occur repeatedly at various points in the process. Fig. 1-1 illustrates the dynamic nature of the nursing process.

Assessment

The nursing process begins with **assessment**—the collection of information about the client's past and current health status and life situation. It is impossible to proceed with nursing care without first obtaining some sense of the client's current status. The subsequent steps in the nursing process are dependent on the availability of accurate information about the client. The extent or depth of assessment may range from being narrowly focused to developing a comprehensive nursing database. For example, in the emergency situation in which a client is found unresponsive in his bed, the nurse takes only a few seconds to assess

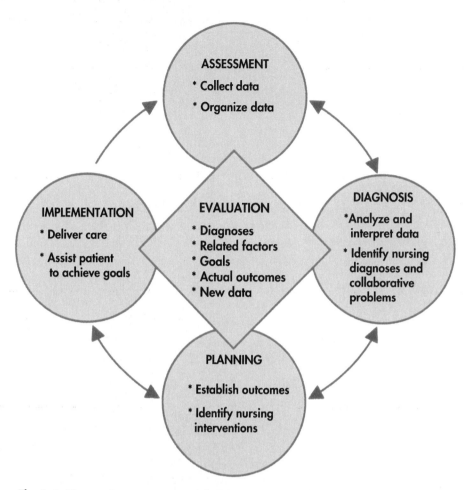

Fig. 1-1 The nursing process. (Modified from Lewis S, Collier I, Heitkemper M: *Medical-surgical nursing: assessment and management of clinical problems,* ed 4, St Louis, 1996, Mosby.)

airway and respiratory status before intervening (that is, calling for help and initiating CPR). No further data are needed prior to beginning these interventions. A more comprehensive assessment is indicated for a client admitted to a long-term care facility following a stroke. Nurses use their clinical judgment to determine the appropriate level of assessment for each client. (See Chapter 2 for a detailed discussion of assessment.)

A simple list of facts collected about a client is not very useful in directing nursing care. What do the facts mean? What client problems do they suggest? The use of a structured assessment framework helps the nurse develop a systematic approach to the collection, organization, and documentation of client data. Such an approach is an important aid in the recognition of significant findings and identification of diagnostic cues. A commonly used approach and the one used in this book is the Functional Health Pattern format developed by Gordon[2] (see Appendix B).

Diagnostic cues are clinically useful facts about the client's status. These cues help to direct additional data collection efforts. Diagnostic cues also suggest possible areas of client strengths and problems. These cues help the nurse begin to make some decisions about client status as the assessment data are collected. As nurses gain experience and become expert clinicians, the ability to draw inferences from diagnostic cues and begin the process of diagnosing occurs simultaneously with the assessment process itself.

Diagnosis

Diagnosis, the second step of the nursing process, assigns meaning to the data collected and organized during assessment. The process of diagnosing enables the nurse to identify specific client responses. These responses are then used as the basis for planning individualized nursing care.

There are two types of problems the nurse can identify: nursing diagnoses and collaborative problems. A **nursing diagnosis** has been defined by the North American Nursing Diagnosis Association (NANDA) as "a clinical judgment about individual, family, or community responses to actual or potential health problems/life processes. Nursing diagnoses provide the basis for selection of nursing interventions to achieve outcomes for which the nurse is accountable."[3] Nursing diagnoses focus on human responses rather than physiologic events or complications. They reflect the component of nursing practice that is independent and for which nurses are professionally accountable. Nursing diagnoses are based on client-specific assessment data, clinical knowledge and experience, and knowledge specific to individual nursing diagnoses. They are written to include a diagnostic label, an etiology, and the defining characteristics (also called signs and symptoms) that support the diagnosis. While the diagnostic labels are standardized, the etiology and specific defining characteristics are unique to each client. The following is an example of a diagnostic statement: *sleep pattern disturbance related to nighttime work schedule and noisy daytime sleep environment as manifested by difficulty remaining asleep and dozing at work.* (Specific guidelines for writing nursing diagnoses are given in Chapter 2.)

Writing nursing diagnoses requires the ability to collect, analyze, and interpret data; apply diagnostic reasoning; and select the most appropriate descriptor (diagnostic label) of the client problem. Just as physicians must differentiate between two similar diagnoses, such as asthma and bronchitis, nurses must be able to differentially diagnose such similar problems as *social isolation* and *diversional activity deficit.* In other words, nurses must make diagnoses that are precise and accurate. A nursing diagnosis is **accurate** when it is consistent with the cues obtained in the client assessment.[4] To make an accurate diagnosis, all cues must be considered in the context of an individual client's situation. The specific cues are then judged to be relevant or irrelevant both as individual cues and as aggregate or interactive cues. Cues that either support or eliminate a particular diagnosis must be examined. Accuracy is achieved when all cues have been thoroughly evaluated, nonrelevant cues have been eliminated and highly relevant ones confirmed, and the data have been examined in a holistic fashion. The characteristics of accuracy of nursing diagnoses as identified by Lunney are listed in Table 1-1.

Writing accurate nursing diagnoses can be one of the more difficult parts of the nursing process. This difficulty is due to the interpretive nature of diagnosing and the complexity of the critical thinking skills involved in the selection of accurate diagnoses. The nurse uses specific nursing knowledge as well as knowledge from the biologic and social sciences and humanities. Mastery of these skills is attained through experience and practice.

The second type of problem the nurse can identify is a collaborative problem. **Collaborative problems** are physiologic complications that require both nursing and medical intervention.[5] The nurse must recognize collaborative problems based on the assessment data collected and knowledge of the physiologic complications of disease processes. The nurse then designs strategies to detect the onset and monitor the course of these problems. The physician prescribes appropriate medical interventions. Collaborative problems include such clinical issues as hypoglycemia, hypoxia, and hypertension.

Planning

The third step in the nursing process is planning. In the **planning** step the nurse thinks carefully about each nursing diagnosis identified. She then considers which nursing actions will be most effective in resolving the diagnosed problems.

TABLE 1-1
Characteristics of Accuracy of Nursing Diagnoses

- The accuracy of a nursing diagnosis is relative to the interactive elements in a client situation.
- The challenge of achieving high levels of accuracy ranges from simple to complex depending on the number of cues, types of cues, and characteristics of cues.
- Accuracy includes the use of supporting and conflicting cues.
- High degrees of accuracy of nursing diagnosis are the result of integrating all of the obtainable cues to make as precise a statement as possible.
- The stringency of achieving accuracy is relative to the situation.
- Low-accuracy diagnoses reflect one or more of the following characteristics:
  Use of unreliable or invalid cues
  Ignorance or misinterpretation of conflicting cues
  Lack of integration of relevant cues for other diagnoses
  Evidence that another diagnosis is more likely
  Lack of agreement with the client or other experts on the phenomena in question

From Lunney M: Accuracy of nursing diagnoses: concept development, *Nursing Diagnosis* 1:1, 1990.

Setting priorities is an important component of planning. A number of diagnoses, as well as collaborative problems, can be identified for most clients. These problems are not all equally significant nor are they equally useful in directing care. The most serious client problems must be quickly identified and treated. Priority problems include emergent and life-threatening/safety situations such as *ineffective airway clearance, risk for violence,* and *potential complication: hemorrhage.* Priority issues may include both nursing diagnoses and collaborative problems.

When no life-threatening problems exist, the nurse uses both professional judgment and the client's evaluation of the importance of each diagnosis to set priorities. Once priorities are determined, the planning process can proceed.

The planning process has two distinct components. The first is the establishment of goals and expected outcomes for each diagnosis. **Goals** are broad, general aims for the client. **Expected outcomes** are more specific objectives related to the goal. Expected outcomes are written as precise and measurable statements that establish the desired client response to care. Achievement of the expected outcomes is used to evaluate the success of the nursing interventions. See the Nursing Diagnosis box below as an example.

NURSING DIAGNOSIS

Constipation related to low dietary fiber intake as manifested by irregular, hard, painful bowel movements twice a week or less

Goal   The client will achieve relief from constipation.

Expected Outcomes

1. Before discharge from the hospital, the client will identify five sources of dietary fiber that she can add to her current diet daily.
2. The client will report including at least three high-fiber foods in her daily diet by her next office visit.
3. The client will report the establishment of a regular bowel pattern with soft, formed, and painless stools by the next office visit.

In the example shown above, the care plan is written to include both the goal and the expected outcomes. It is also acceptable to include only the expected outcomes in the written plan, in which case the goal is implied by the expected outcomes. The latter method is used throughout this text.

Once expected outcomes are established, specific nursing care strategies are designed to help the client achieve these outcomes. Planning identifies interventions that address management, observations or assessments, and client education specific to the nursing diagnosis. Based on the diagnosis of *constipation* and the expected outcomes listed earlier, the following types of nursing interventions would be planned:

1. Review with the client the importance of dietary fiber in preventing constipation.
2. Discuss sources of dietary fiber.
3. Provide a written list of high-fiber foods.
4. Instruct the client to keep a written diet and elimination history so that her fiber intake and elimination pattern can be evaluated at her next office visit.

When establishing expected outcomes and interventions it is important to include the client in the planning. This increases acceptance of the plan by both the client and family. The client must agree with the goals and outcomes and find the interventions acceptable if the plan is to succeed. Table 1-2 displays another example of the planning phase of the nursing process.

The process of planning does not end with the development of an initial plan of care. Planning is an ongoing process that continues as problems are resolved or modified and as additional diagnoses are identified. The goal is to create a plan of care that evolves to reflect the changing client situation.

Implementation

The fourth step of the nursing process is implementation. In the **implementation** step the care plan is put into action through the nursing interventions. **Interventions** are actions the nurse performs to treat the nursing diagnosis. The nurse uses all of her skills, knowledge, and experience, along with the art of nursing, to deliver the planned care and assist the client in achieving the expected outcomes. While providing care the nurse simultaneously performs assessment and collects additional data about the client's status and responses to care. These data are used to determine the status of the current nursing diagnoses and to formulate additional diagnoses if indicated. How the nurse carries out the interventions is just as important as which interventions are implemented. Competence, flexibility, caring, and sensitivity are important elements of good nursing care.

TABLE 1-2

Planning Phase of the Nursing Process

Situation

Mr. Garcia is a 72-year-old man hospitalized with congestive heart failure. His mobility is limited and he spends most of his day in bed. He has moderate (2+) edema of the ankles, feet, legs, sacral area, and hands. He has erythematous areas on his left heel and ankle; the skin is intact but the erythema remains even with relief of pressure (stage I pressure ulcer).

Nursing Diagnosis

Impaired skin integrity related to pressure, edema, and immobility as manifested by erythematous areas on left heel and ankle

Expected Outcomes

1. Decreased redness of skin on left heel and ankle over next 1 to 2 weeks.
2. No breakdown of skin over the feet, ankles, or legs.
3. No new areas of redness over vulnerable areas, including coccyx and other bony prominences.
4. No increase in edema of legs, ankles, or feet.

Interventions

1. Assess skin integrity and edema q 8 h.
2. Cover erythematous areas with a transparent dressing.
3. Pad heels and ankles with foam boots.
4. Place egg-crate mattress on bed.
5. Perform passive ROM exercises to extremities q 4 h.
6. Assist patient in changing position q 2 h.
7. Elevate legs with one pillow while supine or sitting in bed.

Evaluation

Evaluation is the final step in the nursing process. In the **evaluation** stage the client's status and expected outcomes are reviewed. This allows the nurse to determine the extent to which the planned outcomes for each nursing diagnosis have been achieved.

Each diagnosis is evaluated. Important questions to ask about each diagnosis being evaluated include:

1. Is the diagnosis still appropriate or has it been resolved?
2. Does the problem statement or etiology require modification?
3. Are the goals still relevant or do they need modification?
4. Have the expected outcomes been met?
5. Are there data to support additional new diagnoses?

The effectiveness of each intervention in the care plan is also evaluated. For every current nursing diagnosis, the most effective interventions are continued. Nursing actions that have not been effective are deleted from the plan. New interventions are added as needed to support achievement of the expected outcomes.

Let's return to the client with the diagnosis *constipation related to low dietary fiber intake*. To effectively evaluate the nursing interventions, the nurse determines if the client still has pain on defecation and reviews her dietary fiber choices to see if she has indeed included at least three high-fiber foods each day. The client's current bowel elimination pattern must also be assessed. If all of the expected outcomes have been accomplished, the nursing interventions have succeeded. If the expected outcomes have not been achieved, several issues must be explored. Were the goals and outcomes realistic for this client or do they need revision? What are the barriers to attainment of the expected outcomes? Which interventions need to be revised or eliminated and what new interventions may be useful? Were the original etiology and diagnosis accurate? To answer these questions it is necessary to collect additional assessment data. The nursing diagnosis, etiology, goals, expected outcomes, and planned nursing interventions are then revised to reflect the client's current status and needs.

Critical Thinking

The variety and complexity of human responses to health problems and life situations are almost limitless. Therefore nurses must use special cognitive skills, referred to as critical thinking skills, to diagnose and plan interventions to treat client responses.

Critical thinking is a special way of handling information that calls upon all of one's resources—intellect, knowledge, creativity, experience, intuition, and reasoning. Using these resources the nurse generates ideas, considers alternative explanations, draws conclusions, and makes accurate judgments about the client's needs.

Critical thinking is always purposeful and goal directed. Ideas are generated and evaluated, and judgments are made. Critical thinking may be contrasted with "casual" or "random" thinking, which takes place during most of our waking hours. Casual thinking is not goal directed, purposeful, or conclusive even though the mind is active. Critical thinking is always directed toward formulating ideas, conclusions, or diagnoses.

DIAGNOSTIC REASONING

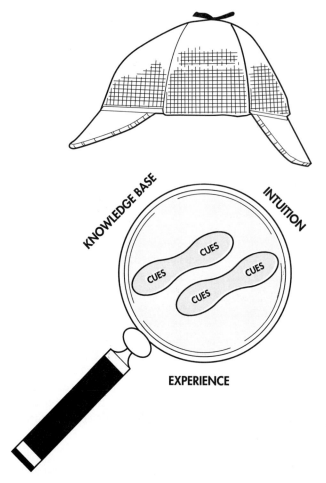

Fig. 1-2 The process of making a nursing diagnosis involves clustering several cues together, making a judgement, and arriving at a nursing diagnosis. This process is similar to the one used by a detective investigating a crime.

Diagnostic reasoning is a specific type of reasoning that uses critical thinking to formulate a nursing diagnosis or identify a collaborative problem (Fig. 1-2). This complex critical thinking process involves the use of one's knowledge base, intuition, and experience to examine and evaluate client cues and identify an accurate nursing diagnosis or collaborative problem.

Relevance to Nursing

Nursing science is becoming increasingly complex as advances occur in the health care field. Because of expansion in knowledge and treatment modalities, the nurse is challenged to integrate technical competence with the art of caring. Meeting this dual challenge requires that the nurse have the ability to think critically at all stages of the nursing process in order to make sound decisions and accurate nursing diagnoses.

The nurse must consistently use a critical thinking approach in making clinical judgments regardless of the practice setting. Important aspects of these judgments are:

1. **Identification of relevant information.** The nurse's assessment must yield specific, sensitive, and important cues. Critical thinking helps to differentiate between important and unimportant client data. Data which are important in one client situation may be unimportant in another. Critical thinking helps the nurse individualize assessment strategies and choose data that are important to a specific client situation. An example of relevant information is the client's statement about why he is seeking health care. Another example is the client's height and weight, which are relevant when evaluating nutritional status.

2. **Consideration of alternatives.** Before making a nursing diagnosis the nurse explores a variety of possible diagnoses. The nurse does not "jump to conclusions" about a diagnosis. By considering alternative diagnoses, the nurse keeps an open mind until the data analysis clearly supports a specific nursing diagnosis. For example, consider the following data:

   1. female client, 5′4″, 182 pounds
   2. 32 years old
   3. reports being highly stressed and overworked
   4. does not exercise.

   Based on these data the nurse considers several alternative nursing diagnoses, including:

   - *altered nutrition: more than body requirements*
   - *ineffective individual coping*
   - *altered health maintenance*

   Additional data must be collected before an accurate diagnosis is chosen. Critical thinking skills help the nurse think through the cues to generate possible diagnoses, identify additional data needed, and consider each proposed diagnosis.
3. **Development of accurate diagnosis.** The diagnostic statement must be consistent with the cues identified in the assessment. The nurse uses critical thinking in considering all the cues in a client situation. It is also important for the nurse to explore conflicting cues. For example, if the client states that he takes his medication as ordered, but the nurse finds more pills left in the bottle than there should be if the client had taken them correctly, there is a conflict between the cues. The nurse must explore the situation further in order to isolate the most accurate data and reach the most accurate diagnosis. Critical thinking also helps the nurse sort through the cues to identify the etiology of the diagnosis identified.
4. **Development of individualized plans of care.** Critical thinking skills are needed to help the nurse develop individualized approaches to client care. This occurs as the nurse works with the client and family to develop expected outcomes for each diagnosis and designs nursing care strategies to facilitate the client's ability to achieve these outcomes. Since every client is unique, it is important to carefully evaluate and individualize a standardized nursing care plan. Diverse interventions may be needed to accomplish the same goals for different clients. To develop ideas about the most appropriate outcomes and care strategies, the nurse must apply knowledge about the individual client, her illness or situation, and her responses. The nurse must then work with the client to refine the plan and evaluate its acceptance by the client and family.
5. **Timely intervention.** The nurse must be able to make decisions rapidly enough to intervene effectively. Critical thinking helps the nurse set priorities and achieve a satisfactory balance between speed and accuracy. For example, a diagnosis such as *ineffective airway clearance* may need to be made quickly as the need for intervention may be urgent. A diagnosis such as *social isolation* does not usually have as high a degree of urgency and could be deferred until more immediate priorities are met and a broad range of supporting cues are identified to confirm the diagnosis.
6. **Evaluation of care.** Nurses must make judgments about the effectiveness of their care. This requires the ability to analyze the client's achievement of each expected outcome as well as the efficacy of each intervention. The nurse must be able to analyze personal behaviors involved in providing care and assisting the client to achieve goals. These activities all require critical thinking skills.

   Critical thinking is used in every step of the nursing process as nurses collect, cluster, and analyze data; formulate nursing diagnoses and collaborative problems; design approaches to client care; and evaluate outcomes. Critical thinking enables the nurse to provide care that is appropriate, individualized, creative, sensitive, comprehensive, and of high quality.

Critical Thinking Strategies

Certain strategies used by the nurse are fundamental features of the critical thinking skills necessary to produce accurate nursing diagnoses. Examples of these strategies include recognizing pertinent, significant data; clarifying, verifying, and validating clinical data; using appropriate resources; using an organized assessment format to obtain the necessary database; and generating multiple diagnostic hypotheses for consideration in the diagnostic process. These strategies will be discussed in detail in Chapter 2.

Characteristics of a Critically Thinking Nurse

The critically thinking nurse exhibits the following specific characteristics (Table 1-3):

1. **Nursing focused.** The critically thinking nurse maintains a clear focus on the domain of nursing—on the human responses of the individual, group, or community to a problem or its treatment. For example, the nursing focus for a client with a fractured femur would include pain

T A B L E   1 - 3
Characteristics of a Critically Thinking Nurse
• Nursing focused • Knowledgeable • Clinically expert • Open minded • Sensitive to interactional issues • Sensitive to contextual issues

management, maintenance of skin integrity, and provision of care required by the client's limited mobility. Nursing care would not focus on what type of pin should be used to stabilize the fracture or what type of anesthesia should be used during surgery.

2. **Knowledgeable.** The critically thinking nurse is able to retrieve defining characteristics from memory, analyze data quickly and methodically, and communicate clearly. This knowledge develops over time and with experience. To develop an adequate knowledge base the nurse should use appropriate references, resources, and consultants to guide practice.

Both novice and expert nurses need to continue to acquire knowledge by reading nursing literature, attending in-service meetings, and attending continuing education programs. In addition, further education through advanced academic preparation in nursing is very valuable in expanding one's knowledge base.

3. **Clinically expert.** Critically thinking nurses use each client encounter to add to their fund of knowledge about human responses. They also examine past experiences for identification of commonalities. For example, the expert nurse would remember that the last time a certain complex of signs and symptoms was seen, the client had a particular nursing diagnosis. Based on her focus, knowledge, and clinical experience, the nurse is able to identify the clinically relevant cues (major defining characteristics), diagnose the problem, and initiate an appropriate plan of nursing care.

4. **Open-minded.** The critically thinking nurse is curious about cues and considers a variety of possible explanations for them. For example, the nurse would not assume that a client's refusal to ambulate following surgery was necessarily due to fear of pain. The nurse's open-mindedness raises questions about other possible reasons for the client's refusal to ambulate. The nurse would carry out further investigation and assessment to clarify the meaning of the client's refusal to ambulate. The critically thinking nurse would consider a variety of possible reasons, including fatigue, fear of falling, not wanting to be seen publicly while looking "unpresentable," or a cultural belief that after surgery one should "rest." Failure to remain open-minded can result in diagnostic errors.

5. **Sensitive to interactional and contextual issues.** The critically thinking nurse is sensitive to the dynamics of interactions between the nurse and client, the nurse-client-family, or the client and others. The nurse recognizes that a wide range of interactions are possible among people. The nurse learns to assess the complexity of peoples' interactions and recognizes how these interactions affect clients. To accomplish this the nurse uses the tools of effective communication and a basic knowledge of human behavior.

The nurse must also consider the context (circumstances, conditions, or setting) in which the data are presented. For example, the client's behavior may change in the privacy of her home as compared with the hospital environment. This can influence the validity (confirmation or substantiation) and reliability (ability to obtain the same results on separate occasions) of the assessment data collected and can also have an impact on the client's responses to care. Another example of context has to do with the circumstances in which care is provided, such as routine versus emergency situations. In an emergency situation, priorities of life and safety take precedence over all other issues. The nurse focuses on those cues that have a bearing on the client's most important body functions—airway, breathing, and circulation. The nurse must recognize also that client responses to an emergency may not be typical of the client's usual response patterns and will need to be reevaluated after the crisis is over. The nurse's consideration of these contextual variables will affect data collection as well as data analysis, diagnosis, and intervention.

Summary

The five steps of the nursing process are assessment, diagnosis, planning, implementation, and evaluation. This process provides a framework for the identification and treatment of client problems. The nursing process is an ongoing and interactive cycle that results in flexible, individualized, and dynamic nursing care for all clients. Assessment is the foundation of the process and leads to the identification of both nursing diagnoses and collaborative problems. Nursing diagnoses provide the primary focus for the development of client-specific plans of nursing care. The planning process allows for the individualization of client goals and nursing care. Implementation is the provision of nursing actions to treat each diagnosis. Ongoing evaluation determines the degree of success in achieving the client's goals and the continued relevance of each nursing diagnosis and collaborative problem.

The implementation of the nursing process requires complex clinical and diagnostic knowledge and the application of critical thinking skills. Learning and applying these skills is a challenge for the novice and requires a great deal of practice.

Guidelines for Writing Nursing Diagnoses

Differentiating Medical Diagnoses, Nursing Diagnoses, and Collaborative Problems

There are three types of problems that can be identified for a client—medical diagnoses, nursing diagnoses, and collaborative problems. The nurse's responsibility is to recognize nursing diagnoses as those problems that can be diagnosed and treated independently by professional nurses. An important part of the process of making a nursing diagnosis is determining that the problem is in fact a nursing diagnosis and not a medical diagnosis or a collaborative problem.

The major difference between a medical and a nursing diagnosis is the focus of practice. Medical practice is focused on the diagnosis and treatment of illness; nursing practice is focused on the diagnosis and treatment of human responses to health problems/life processes. There are also legal parameters that determine boundaries of practice. These parameters are outlined in the professional practice acts of the respective disciplines. A look at the primary goals of nursing and medicine helps in differentiating between them (Table 2-1).

Collaborative problems overlap the two disciplines. These problems are ones for which both nursing and medicine prescribe treatments.

Medical Diagnosis

A **medical diagnosis** is the label given to the disease or syndrome a person has or is suspected of having. The physician uses scientific and skilled methods to establish the cause and nature of a person's illness. The diagnosis of medical problems is accomplished by analyzing the history of the disease process, performing a physical examination, and evaluating results of diagnostic studies. The medical diagnosis is used to provide a logical basis for medical treatment. It is accepted by the medical profession as an efficient way to describe a complex of signs and symptoms for which the physician is responsible for providing medical treatment. A medical diagnosis is always related to pathology, whether it is organ pathology (myocardial infarction or glomerulonephritis, for instance) or psychopathology (schizophrenia or depression).

The work of defining medical diagnoses has been evolving over the past two centuries. In addition to guiding medical practice, a medical diagnosis is used for other reasons. For example, medical diagnoses are used by the United States government to identify the diagnosis-related groups (DRGs) that are the basis for the prospective federal payment system, which reimburses for medical care for Medicare clients. Also, diagnoses are grouped in an International Classification of Diseases of Medicine (ICDM), compiled and revised by the World Health Organization every 10 years.

T A B L E 2 - 1	
Comparison of Primary Goals: **Nursing and Medicine**	
NURSING	**MEDICINE**
Determines responses to health problems, level of wellness, and need for assistance	Determines cause of illness or injury
Provides physical care, emotional care, teaching, guidance, and counseling	Provides medical treatments and surgery
Interventions aimed at assisting the client to meet own needs	Interventions aimed at preventing and curing injury or illness

From Lewis S, Collier I, Heitkemper P: *Medical-surgical nursing: assessment and management of clinical problems,* ed 4, St Louis, 1996, Mosby.

This classification system has many uses, among which are collection of data related to morbidity, mortality, incidence, and prevalence of different diseases.

The nurse is not responsible for making a medical diagnosis, but is expected to understand what the medical diagnosis is: that is, she should understand the signs and symptoms, pathophysiology, and treatment ordered by physicians. Nurses are also responsible for the recognition of deviations from normal health patterns that require referral to a physician. The nurse must recognize the presence of nursing diagnoses and collaborative problems associated with medical diagnoses.

Nursing Diagnosis

A **nursing diagnosis** is defined on p. 5 as "a clinical judgment about individual, family, or community responses to actual or potential health problems/life processes. Nursing diagnoses provide the basis for selection of nursing interventions to achieve outcomes for which the nurse is accountable."[3] A nursing diagnosis is a judgment made by the nurse after rigorous analysis and synthesis of assessment data. Thus a nursing diagnosis is the result of an assessment of the total person-environment interaction reflecting client responses that are amenable to independent nursing intervention.[6] The nursing diagnosis statement describes both the response of the client (diagnostic label) and factors contributing to that response (etiology) as well as associated signs and symptoms.

The nursing diagnosis frequently results from the client's response to his disease process. For example,

a client may have the medical diagnosis of chronic obstructive pulmonary disease (COPD). The nursing diagnosis, however, would relate to how the client responds to COPD (for example, *activity intolerance related to imbalance between oxygen supply and demand as manifested by SOB with exertion and increased heart rate after ambulating*). The nurse initiates interventions for treatment of this nursing diagnosis. Interventions could include assisting the client to increase activity level gradually or teaching energy conservation methods for activities of daily living.

A number of other terms or situations are not nursing diagnoses but are often mislabeled as such. These include:

Medical pathology (anemia)
Diagnostic tests or studies (complete blood cell count)
Equipment (indwelling catheter)
Signs (restlessness)
Symptoms (nausea)
Surgical procedures (exploratory laparotomy)
Treatments (dressing change)
Therapeutic goals (should increase calorie intake)
Nursing problems (difficult to turn)
Therapeutic needs (needs more rest)
Staff problems (Mr. Jones is too demanding)

Since 1973, the North American Nursing Diagnosis Association (NANDA) has been working on developing a taxonomy to classify nursing diagnoses. This organization originally represented nurses from Canada and the United States. Today there are members from many other nations. The original goals of identifying nursing diagnoses and developing a taxonomy continue to be the focus of this organization. NANDA was recognized by the American Nurses Association as the body to be utilized for the development, review, and approval of nursing diagnoses. Presently there are 128 nursing diagnoses accepted by NANDA for clinical use and testing. These diagnoses are organized into the Taxonomy I–Revised using the human response patterns framework developed by NANDA.[3]

Another classification of nursing diagnoses is the Omaha Classification Scheme, which identifies "domains, problems, and signs/symptoms addressed by nurses in the community health setting."[7] In addition, several other nursing specialty groups such as the critical care, psychiatric, and orthopedic nursing associations, have been working on developing and classifying nursing diagnoses. The American Nurses Association supported further taxonomy development by NANDA in 1988 and urged nursing groups to unite in this effort.

Collaborative Problems

The **bifocal clinical practice model** was introduced by Carpenito in 1983.[8] This model identifies the two clinical situations in which nurses intervene—one as primary provider through the appropriate nursing diagnosis and the other as collaborator with other disciplines. **Collaborative problems** are certain physiologic complications that nurses monitor to detect onset or changes in status. Examples of collaborative problems are:

- *Potential complication: paralytic ileus*
- *Potential complication: increased intracranial pressure*

Nurses manage collaborative problems using both physician-prescribed and nurse-prescribed interventions. The focus of nursing care in collaborative problems is to recognize and minimize the complications associated with the health problem.[5]

All collaborative problem statements begin with the phrase "potential complication" or "PC." This phrase implies that the nurse is responsible for carrying out relevant medical directives as well as determining appropriate nursing interventions. The focus for the nurse is to reduce the severity of complications or to prevent them from occurring. When the label "potential complication" is used, the client may be either currently experiencing the complication (for instance, hemorrhaging) or may be at risk for experiencing the complication (for instance, not currently bleeding but at risk because of a low platelet count). In either case the collaborative problem statement would be *potential complication: hemorrhage.*

In order to identify collaborative problems, the nurse needs to know the range of complications that can result from diseases or treatment measures. Assessment for collaborative problems requires the nurse to examine the status of the client problem using knowledge and experience about the medical diagnosis to anticipate or predict those complications that the client is likely to experience. As the nurse's knowledge base and experience increase, accurate identification of these problems becomes easier. Until the nurse is an expert clinician, she needs to use reference books to aid in the recognition of these complications.

Case Example

The following example will illustrate the difference between nursing diagnoses, medical diagnoses, and collaborative problems.

Mr. Williams, 20 years old, is admitted to the hospital for the fourth time with the medical diagnosis of lymphoma. The physician writes the following medical orders:

- vital signs q 8 h
- bedrest
- regular diet
- chest tube to wall suction with 25 cm pressure
- MS Contin 30 mg po q 4 h prn pain

The nurse will implement these medical orders, as well as collect additional data and organize it using the functional health pattern framework.

Health Perception/Health Management Pattern

1. Aware of deterioration in his condition
2. Expects to have relief of difficulty in breathing from the chest tube
3. Does not expect to be cured of his lymphoma

Nutritional/Metabolic Pattern

1. Complains of nausea and painful mouth as a result of side effects of chemotherapy
2. Eats small amounts of yogurt and ice cream three or four times a day
3. Drinks four glasses of water a day
4. Weight loss of three pounds a week for past two months
5. Skin dry, intact
6. Ulcerations of oral cavity
7. WBC 3500/μL (normal: 5,000 to 10,000)

Elimination Pattern

1. Bowel movements hard and q 2 days
2. Urine clear, yellow, and four or five times a day

Activity/Exercise Pattern

1. Reports unable to do much for himself, gets very short of breath and starts coughing when active
2. Needs assistance in getting to the bathroom
3. Does not dress, stays in pajamas during the day
4. Is able to hold a spoon and a glass
5. Right chest tube connected to water seal drainage
6. Crackles over both lung fields
7. Coughing occasionally produces white sputum
8. Oxygen saturation 86%

Sleep/Rest Pattern

1. Sleep interrupted by coughing during the night
2. Sleeps only for short periods (15 to 20 minutes)
3. Naps frequently throughout the day
4. Feels tired all the time

Cognitive/Perceptual Pattern

1. Complains of pain in chest all the time
2. Uses MS Contin at home
3. Has had to increase dosage during the past two weeks
4. Gets good pain relief from this medication
5. Alert but appears somnolent
6. Communicates infrequently

Self-Perception/Self-Concept Pattern

1. Expresses concern about having a chest tube again
2. Feels like nothing is helping to make him get better

Role/Relationship Pattern

1. Lives with his family, who are very supportive
2. Mother provides around-the-clock care for him at home
3. Friends come to visit him occasionally

Sexuality/Reproductive Pattern

1. Sexually active with girlfriend prior to illness onset one year ago

Coping/Stress Tolerance Pattern

1. Appears sad all the time
2. Expresses losing hope that he will get well
3. Worries about his family and how they will do if he dies
4. Uses prayer and talking to his mother to deal with his concerns

Value/Belief Pattern

1. Minister comes in daily to pray with him
2. Expresses doubt about the effectiveness of the chest tube and chemotherapy

Based on this data, nursing diagnoses are:

- *Altered oral mucous membrane related to effects of chemotherapy as manifested by complaint of painful mouth and ulcerations of the mouth*
- *Sleep pattern disturbance related to coughing and pain as manifested by observed frequent napping and expression of tiredness*
- *Altered nutrition: less than body requirements related to oral pain, nausea, and fatigue as manifested by weight loss of three pounds a week*
- *Hopelessness related to repeated complications of disease as manifested by apathy, verbalization about chest tube, decreased interaction and infrequent communication*

The nursing diagnoses in this situation address the complexity of this individual's response to the disease and its treatment. The nursing diagnoses also change as the client's responses change. The medical diagnosis, however, does not change.

The collaborative problems in this example are:

- *PC: hypoxemia*
- *PC: immunodeficiency*

Clearly, both nursing and medical interventions are required to treat these conditions. Delegated medical functions using protocols or standing orders may be part of the nurse's role in treating collaborative problems. This requires an adequate knowledge base and clinical expertise to make safe clinical judgments. The nurse also plans interventions to prevent these potential complications and to treat them if they should occur.

Writing Nursing Diagnoses

Up to this point, the focus of this book has been on the theoretical bases for nursing diagnosis. It is now time to learn the fundamental principles relating to writing the nursing diagnosis statement.

Basic Structure

There is a basic structure or format to writing a nursing diagnosis statement. The names of the various parts can be confusing, as the literature uses several different names for the same component part. Table 2-2 describes the different terms that are used for the parts of a nursing diagnosis statement. This book uses the terms *diagnostic label, related factors,* and *defining characteristics.*

TABLE 2-2
Different Terms Used in Writing Diagnostic Statements
Diagnostic Label
Problem
Label
Title
Related Factors
Contributing factors
Risk factors
Etiology
Defining Characteristics
Signs and symptoms
Clinical manifestations

Diagnostic Label
What Is the Problem?

The **diagnostic label,** the initial word or words in the diagnostic statement, is the descriptive phrase that clearly and concisely states the client's response to a health problem/life process. Generally the label is taken from the NANDA list of approved nursing diagnoses. However, because nursing diagnosis is still in a developmental stage, not all client responses have been clearly defined. Because of this, when the nurse in clinical practice identifies a response that is not currently on the NANDA list, a new diagnosis may be developed to cover the problem. For example, *dysfunctional alcohol use,* not currently a NANDA-approved diagnosis, might be useful in certain settings when significant signs and symptoms are present. If the nurse has trouble selecting a specific nursing diagnosis, either NANDA-approved or an original one, it may be a clue that there is not yet sufficient data for making a clinical judgment. In this case the nurse would collect additional assessment data to clarify the appropriate nursing diagnosis.

Nursing literature contains non-NANDA diagnoses that have been found to be clinically useful. For instance, Carpenito discusses *grieving* as a natural human response to an actual or perceived loss.[5] Gordon presents information on *pain self-management deficit* in her manual.[9] Neither of these two diagnoses are NANDA-approved. Both of these authors describe numerous non–NANDA-approved diagnoses that clinicians may find useful in their practice.

Related Factors
What Are the Causes of or Contributing Factors to the Problem?

This part of the nursing diagnosis statement contains a brief description of the probable cause of (etiology) or factors that have contributed to the problem. This statement is generally preceded by the phrase "related to."

Carpenito identifies four categories of related factors:[5]

1. Pathophysiologic (biologic or psychologic), such as loss of body part or cognitive impairment
2. Treatment related, such as traction/casts or painful treatment
3. Situational (environmental, personal), such as stress, wet body surface, or interrupted sleep pattern
4. Maturational, such as decreased metabolic needs or loss of skin elasticity

The selection of accurate related factors is of critical importance when writing the diagnostic statement. This is because it is the related factors or etiology that direct nursing interventions. Interventions for these factors should be within the realm of independent nursing practice. Consequently, medical diagnoses should not be used as a related factor in writing a nursing diagnosis. The unofficial position taken by the Diagnosis Review Committee of NANDA is that "if you think of etiologic factors as being the focus of nursing intervention, then it would probably be conceptually inadvisable to cite a medical diagnosis as an etiology because it becomes a focus of nursing treatment."[10]

As can be seen, confusion and incongruencies abound regarding the use of medical diagnoses as related factors. The position taken by the authors of this text and used in the case studies is that a medical diagnosis is generally not a specific enough etiology to be useful in planning care. For example, *impaired physical mobility related to multiple sclerosis* gives no direction for nursing interventions. Whereas, *impaired physical mobility related to lower limb weakness* gives direction to the nurse for planning appropriate interventions. If a medical diagnosis will clarify the related factors, it can be added to the diagnostic statement with the phrase "secondary to." For example, the inclusion of the medical diagnosis in the nursing diagnosis *impaired physical mobility related to lower limb weakness secondary to multiple sclerosis* definitely clarifies the etiology.

When appropriate, the **underlying pathophysiologic process** of a disease can be used as a related factor. For example, *impaired tissue integrity related to low hemoglobin count, prolonged bed rest, and ineffective immune response* is preferable to *impaired tissue integrity related to anemia, prolonged bed rest, and AIDS.* Based on education and experience, the nurse can plan interventions appropriate for the pathophysiologic process. Because the nurse knows that a low hemoglobin count can compromise tissue oxygenation, the plan would call for frequent turning. Because an ineffective immune response puts the client at risk for infection, the plan would include meticulous wound care. Other examples might be the use of increased metabolic rate rather than hyperthyroidism, abnormally thick mucous secretions rather than cystic fibrosis, and paralysis of the facial nerve rather than Bell's palsy.

Defining Characteristics
How Do I Know This Problem Is Present?

The third part of the diagnostic statement consists of the defining characteristics. **Defining characteristics** are the subjective and objective data that lead the nurse to identify a particular problem. This book uses major and minor characteristics as identified by NANDA. When a particular cluster of defining characteristics is present, it suggests a particular nursing diagnosis to the nurse.

Defining characteristics are generally separated into major and minor defining characteristics. **Major defining characteristics** are critical indicators of a problem and are present 80% to 100% of the time when the problem is present. Research has indicated that major characteristics are present in most clients for whom a particular diagnosis is appropriate. The major defining characteristics are not present when a particular nursing diagnosis is not present. **Minor defining characteristics** are supporting indicators of a problem and are present 50% to 79% of the time when the problem is present.

Not all NANDA diagnoses have been clinically tested to establish the major and minor defining characteristics. Carpenito uses a "consensus of experts" approach to differentiate between major and minor defining characteristics that have not been established by research.[5] McFarland and McFarlane caution against using major and minor defining characteristics in establishing the validity of a particular nursing diagnosis.[11] They contend that "differentiating critical defining characteristics from supporting characteristics at this stage of the art and science of nursing diagnosis should be considered developmental because there is little research on which to base such differentiation."[11] Gordon uses the terms *major* and *critical* interchangeably when discussing characteristics that must be present to make a diagnosis. The presence of supporting or minor characteristics support or confirm the diagnosis and increase the nurse's confidence that a correct judgment has been made.[2]

There are times when a defining characteristic is so specific to a diagnosis that its presence ensures the accuracy of the diagnosis. For instance, if a client states that she is in pain, this single defining characteristic is satisfactory for assigning the diagnosis of *pain*.

In general, however, the nurse is cautioned against using only one defining characteristic as the sole criterion on which to select a particular nursing diagnosis. The accuracy of a diagnosis is improved when several defining characteristics, both major and minor, are present. For instance, the presence of multiple cues— agitation, significant increase in vital signs, cyanosis, diaphoresis, and decreased level of consciousness when removed from the ventilator—give assurance that the nursing diagnosis of *dysfunctional ventilatory weaning response* is accurate.

Gordon provides structural and functional guidelines that assist in the formulation of a diagnostic statement.[2] These guidelines include the following

1. The nursing diagnosis describes a dysfunctional or potentially dysfunctional pattern using accepted diagnostic labels.
2. The relationship between the diagnostic categories (label) describing the problem and etiologic (related) factors is indicated by "R/T" or the words "related to."
3. Both the problem (label) and etiology (related factors) refer to distinct clusters of signs and symptoms. The observed signs and symptoms contain the critical defining characteristics for the problem (label) and etiologic (related) factors.
4. Structure of the problem (label) and etiologic (related) factors are concise and clear and include the recommended specifications such as levels and acuity (for example, *self-care deficit: feeding or activity intolerance: level IV).*
5. The etiologic (related) factors or critical risk factors for a potential problem can be predicted to change with nursing intervention, and the change can be predicted to resolve the problem.
6. The problem (label) and etiologic (related) factors are written without ambiguous or highly value-laden words and in legally advisable terms.

Types of Nursing Diagnoses

The exact form or structure of a nursing diagnosis statement depends on its type: actual, risk, possible, syndrome, or wellness (Table 2-3). The components of the different types of nursing diagnoses are listed in Table 2-4.

Actual Nursing Diagnoses

An **actual nursing diagnosis** is a judgment that is clinically validated by the presence of major defining characteristics. It indicates that sufficient assessment

T A B L E   2 - 3
Types of Nursing Diagnoses

- Actual
- Risk
- Possible
- Syndrome
- Wellness

Components of Different Types of Nursing Diagnosis Statements

	DIAGNOSTIC LABEL	RELATED FACTORS	DEFINING CHARACTERISTICS
Actual	✓	✓	✓
Risk	✓	✓	
Possible	✓	✓	
Syndrome	✓		
Wellness	✓		

data are available to establish the nursing diagnosis. It reflects a response the client is experiencing that needs nursing intervention. An actual nursing diagnosis usually contains all three elements of a diagnostic statement—diagnostic label, related factors, and defining characteristics. An example of an actual nursing diagnosis is *anticipatory grieving* (diagnostic label) *related to expected loss of sports scholarship and normal appearance* (related factors) *as manifested by expressed distress at impending lower limb amputation, refusal to eat, and inability to sleep* (defining characteristics).

There are times when only the diagnostic label and related factors are included for an actual diagnosis. When the defining characteristics are readily apparent in the chart or client record, it is not always necessary to repeat them when writing the nursing diagnosis statement. If, however, the defining characteristics are difficult to extract from existing data or are known only to the examining nurse, it is better to include them as the third part of the diagnostic statement.

Risk Nursing Diagnoses

As defined by NANDA, a **risk nursing diagnosis** describes "human responses to health conditions/life precesses which may develop in a vulnerable individual, family, or community."[3] The main issue in establishing a risk diagnosis is vulnerability. The client must be at increased vulnerability for a risk diagnosis to be accurate. A risk diagnosis suggests the presence of risk factors that contribute to increased vulnerability. The nurse draws on knowledge and experience to identify risk factors.

There are many nursing interventions that are considered standard and basic to the care of all clients, regardless of their health problems. For instance, the nurse would consider the need to prevent infection, maintain adequate nutrition, and foster regular elimination in all clients. These basic interventions form the basis of care for all clients and are not usually included in a care plan without a reason. However, the at risk client is considered to be more vulnerable than the average client for the development of a particular problem. For example, although all surgical clients are considered to be at risk for infection, this diagnosis would not routinely be made for the general surgical client. If, however, a diabetic client had surgery, the diagnosis of *risk for infection* would be made. For the at risk client, the primary nursing interventions are directed at the prevention of the problem by specific, planned nursing interventions. The goal of nursing interventions is that the problem never develop.

When writing a risk nursing diagnosis, the diagnostic label is always preceded by the words *risk for*. The related factors are risk factors that the nurse recognizes as making this particular client more vulnerable to experience the problem. Defining characteristics are not used in the diagnostic statement because they are not currently present. However, the nurse, aware of the defining characteristics through education and experience, is alert to their occurrence. Should defining characteristics become apparent, the risk diagnosis would become an actual diagnosis.

An example of this type of diagnosis can be seen in the following case.

Mrs. Martinez is an 82-year-old woman four hours post total hip replacement surgery. She had a spinal anesthetic, is on bed rest for 24 hours, and is receiving patient-controlled analgesia. Her age is the factor that increases her risk. An appropriate nursing diagnosis for this client would be *risk for ineffective airway clearance related to advanced age, immobility, anesthesia, and analgesia.* Note that there are no defining characteristics in the diagnosis because no signs or symptoms of this problem are yet evident. Hopefully, excellent nursing care will prevent the occurrence of the problem. As this client becomes more mobile and requires less analgesia, the diagnosis would no longer be appropriate and would be dropped from the list.

Possible Nursing Diagnoses

A **possible nursing diagnosis** describes a suspected problem for which there are insufficient data currently available. This type of diagnosis is tentative until additional data confirm it as an actual diagnosis or until the absence of relevant cues eliminates it as a diagnostic possibility.

A possible nursing diagnosis is written as a two-part statement. The first part of the statement includes the nursing diagnosis preceded by the word *possible*. The second part of the statement contains the related factors that led the nurse to suspect the diagnosis. An example of this type of statement might be *possible body image disturbance related to physical changes associated with mastectomy*. Without further information, the nurse is uncertain whether the client's reluctance to assist with her dressing change is due to distress over loss of her breast and size of the incision or because she is uncertain how to do the procedure. Further assessment would clarify the validity of this diagnosis.

There are three different outcomes that may be the result of a possible nursing diagnosis.

1. The nurse may obtain sufficient data from additional focused assessment to change the diagnosis from a possible nursing diagnosis to an actual nursing diagnosis.
2. The nurse may obtain sufficient data from additional focused assessment to confirm the client's risk status and change the possible nursing diagnosis to a risk nursing diagnosis.
3. The assessment may fail to confirm the presence of an actual or risk diagnosis because of the lack of major defining characteristics or risk factors. The possible diagnosis would be eliminated completely at this time.

Additional data are necessary to reach any of these three outcomes. When a possible nursing diagnosis is identified, collection of additional data is a key intervention.

Syndrome Nursing Diagnoses

A **syndrome nursing diagnosis** is a diagnostic label given to a distinct cluster of nursing diagnoses that almost always go together and present a specific clinical picture. The use of a syndrome diagnosis is a useful, meaningful, and efficient way to describe a complex problem without having to document each component of the problem as a distinct nursing diagnosis.

When writing a syndrome diagnosis, only the diagnostic label of the syndrome is used. Currently, there are three NANDA-approved syndrome diagnoses—

T A B L E   2 - 5
Nursing Diagnoses Associated with Disuse Syndrome
• *Risk for constipation* • *Risk for altered respiratory function* • *Risk for infection* • *Risk for activity intolerance* • *Risk for injury* • *Impaired physical mobility* • *Risk for altered thought processes* • *Risk for body image disturbance* • *Risk for powerlessness* • *Risk for impaired tissue integrity*

rape trauma syndrome, disuse syndrome, and *relocation stress syndrome*. The diagnostic label contains the primary etiologic factor and does not need to be repeated. For instance, it would be redundant to write *rape trauma syndrome related to recent experience of rape* or *disuse syndrome related to immobility*. The defining characteristics tend to represent a cluster of other nursing diagnoses. Table 2-5 illustrates the actual or risk nursing diagnoses clustered under *disuse syndrome*.

McCourt provides an excellent summary of the common characteristics of syndrome nursing diagnoses:

1. A syndrome diagnosis represents a cluster of nursing diagnoses.
2. The label gives a clue to the cause.
3. Syndrome diagnoses have intermediate and long-term phases.
4. Syndrome diagnoses have emotional, social, and physical components.
5. Syndrome diagnoses represent complex clinical conditions that require expert nursing assessment and expert nursing interventions.[12]

Wellness Nursing Diagnoses

The ANA **Social Policy Statement** states that nursing addresses both sick and well persons and promotes health.[1] This mandate clearly establishes nursing's responsibility to look at wellness promotion. Dimensions of wellness that are useful for nurses to consider include physical fitness, nutritional awareness, stress management, environmental sensitivity, and self-responsibility.[13]

Within the language of nursing diagnosis, the need for nursing to promote higher levels of wellness is addressed through wellness diagnoses. NANDA defines a wellness diagnosis as "a clinical judgment about an individual, group, or community in transition from a specific level of wellness to a higher level of wellness."[3] A wellness diagnosis is used when a client is interested in pursuing optimal health. Carpenito gives good direction in the development of wellness nursing diagnoses.[5] She suggests the following actions:

1. Following completion of a functional health screening assessment, the nurse must decide if a problem is present in any of the functional health patterns. If a problem is identified, the nurse should complete a focused assessment and develop a nursing care plan based on an actual, risk, or possible nursing diagnosis.

2. If no problem is identified, the nurse must then decide if additional planning is appropriate. If not, the conclusion is made that the client is managing effectively in a particular pattern. This conclusion can then be used as a client strength and incorporated into the plan of care for an altered function. If there is indication that it is appropriate (either from the client's request or the nurse's judgment) to assist the client to achieve a higher level of wellness, then a wellness diagnosis can be made.

3. Once the assessment conclusion is made, the nursing diagnosis can be formulated. If the conclusion is that the client desires to move to a higher level of wellness, the nursing diagnosis statement is written as *potential for enhanced _____* . The diagnosis is made specific by adding a descriptor. An example of this type of diagnostic statement might be *potential for enhanced physical fitness*.

Summary

Nurses identify two types of client problems—nursing diagnoses and collaborative problems. Nurses intervene in three types of client problems—nursing diagnoses, collaborative problems, and medical diagnoses. The nurse must be able to differentiate between these types of client problems. Once a nursing diagnosis is identified, it is important that the nurse write a diagnostic statement in the accepted format.

Careful attention to each component of the diagnostic statement—the label, the related factors, and the defining characteristics—increases diagnostic accuracy. Accuracy in writing nursing diagnoses comes with study and practice. If the nurse uses the diagnostic reasoning process and the basic rules for writing a nursing diagnosis, the result will be appropriate nursing interventions leading to desirable client outcomes.

The Process of Making an Accurate Nursing Diagnosis

Diagnostic Process

The diagnostic reasoning process has many similarities to **information processing theory,** described in psychology and used in many other disciplines.[14] The steps in information processing theory are :[15]

1. Client encounter; gather cues
2. Infer relationships among cues; cluster cues (identify general problems)
3. Propose diagnostic hypotheses
4. Perform a focused assessment and hypothesis testing
5. Make a diagnosis

From the information processing theory, a model can be developed that works well for nursing. The diagnostic process model used in this book is depicted in Fig. 3-1. There are three main differences between the information processing theory and the diagnostic process model used in this book. The diagnostic process model uses:

1. Two levels of data clustering
2. Validation of the nursing diagnosis
3. Development of an accurate diagnostic statement

Each of the case studies depicts the application of the diagnostic process model.

Collection of Assessment Data

The process of developing an accurate nursing diagnosis begins with the collection of assessment data. The nurse uses critical thinking during the assessment process to judge what and how much information to collect and what methods and tools are appropriate for data collection. Once the assessment information is collected, the nurse must then evaluate the reliability of the data, judge their relevancy, analyze them for meaning, and decide if additional data are needed.

Purpose of Assessment

Assessment is the nursing activity that initiates the nursing process. The two primary purposes of assessment are to provide a set of systematically collected data that describe the client's response to a health problem or life situation and to identify client strengths and limitations. Additional purposes of assessment include:

* Initiation of the nursing process by providing information basic to the remaining steps of the nursing process
* Identification of needs and services essential for achieving outcome criteria

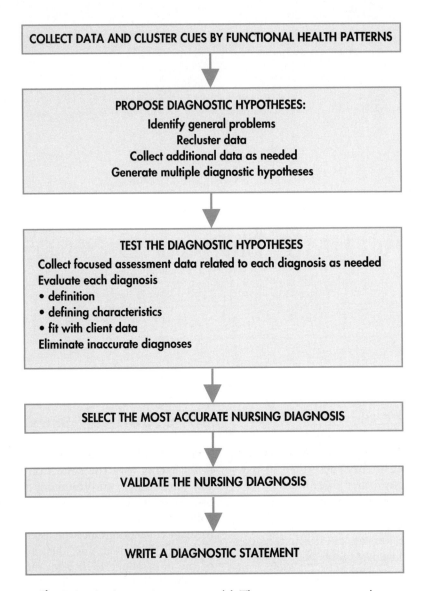

Fig. 3-1 The diagnostic process model. The nurse uses a systematic reasoning approach to develop accurate diagnosis.

- Provision of client-specific information to other health care providers
- Provision of ongoing information to evaluate the effectiveness of nursing interventions
- Legal validation that client assessment has been carried out as mandated by state Nurse Practice Acts and Standards of Practice

The process of client assessment is a dynamic, fluid nursing activity that builds with each client encounter. Generally, assessment begins when the client first enters the health care system, regardless of the setting. For instance, the nurse could have her first encounter with a client on a home visit following a hospitalization, or the initial assessment could involve an admission physical before surgery in a day surgery unit or hospital setting. The important concept is that assessment is an ongoing process closely tied to the client's status. As the client's status changes, there is a need for additional assessment. As assessment data change, the nursing care plan must also change.

Types of Data

There are two types of assessment data—subjective and objective. These data are cues used by the nurse to formulate nursing diagnoses and collaborative problems.

Subjective data are phenomena that are experienced directly by the client. These data, also called **symptoms,** can only be recounted to the nurse by the client. Symptoms such as weakness and fatigue are examples of events that are not generally observable or measurable by the nurse. In order to elicit this information, the nurse could ask the client, "What are your symptoms?" Some symptoms such as shortness of breath may be validated by the nurse by direct observation (for example, client states feeling short of breath and nurse observes flaring nostrils, use of accessory muscles, and diaphoresis). If there appears to be an inconsistency between the client's verbal account of a symptom and an observed behavior (for example, client states feeling nauseated but nurse observes client eating a large meal), additional observation may be necessary. The quality, accuracy, and amount of subjective data collected are often dependent upon the nurse's communication skills and interviewing techniques.

Objective data are phenomena that can be observed or measured. Blood pressure, results of laboratory studies, and the findings of a physical examination are examples of objective data. These types of data can be verified by another examiner. Although objective data are supposed to be free of bias, it is important for the nurse to be aware that personal emotions, prejudices, preconceptions, and lack of knowledge could affect the analysis of the data, making it less objective.

An objective indicator of a health problem is called a **sign.** Signs are usually gathered by observation and examination. Fever, drainage, tachycardia, and orthostatic hypotension are examples of observable or measurable signs indicating health problems.

Objective data might be found in the chart, noted during a physical examination, determined by diagnostic studies, or obtained by other health care providers. The nurse is not responsible for directly providing all objective data.

Organization of Data

The nurse gathers large amounts of data about a particular client over the span of a nurse-client relationship. It would be extremely difficult to sort out the meaning of these data without some method of organization. An organizational framework particularly useful to nurses that examines all areas of client responses has been developed by Gordon and is called **functional health patterns.** This framework guides both the collecting and recording of data. It provides an excellent way to organize data. Appendix A lists the 11 patterns that make up the functional health pattern format and the type of information contained in each pattern.

The functional health patterns provide a holistic view of the client by describing "certain functional patterns that contribute to their health, quality of life, and achievement of human potential."[2] Use of the functional health pattern framework aids the nurse in organizing data, evaluating the client's health, and formulating accurate nursing diagnoses.

The patterns are interrelated, interactive, and interdependent.[2] Because of this, many or all patterns need to be assessed in most situations. For example, Ms. Smith relates that she eats a diet low in fiber and drinks very little fluid (nutrition/metabolic pattern). While these are clinically relevant cues, they are insufficient to diagnose a problem. The client further relates that she takes a laxative periodically since she is very irregular and has hard, dry stools that are painful to pass (elimination pattern). She also indicates that she gets very little exercise since she has limited mobility as a result of arthritis (activity/exercise pattern). Within the elimination pattern the nurse will identify this client's general problem of constipation. Within the other two patterns the nurse will identify possible related factors for this problem—low fiber and fluid intake and immobility.

Types of Assessment

There are three types of assessment—comprehensive, focused, and screening—that the nurse can use to obtain initial or ongoing data about a client. The use of a particular type of assessment is a clinical judgment. The type of assessment used depends upon the client's condition, amount of time available, purpose of the encounter, probable length of relationship, and the nurse's expertise.

Comprehensive Assessment

A **comprehensive assessment** is the most complete type of assessment a nurse would perform on a client. In this assessment a complete nursing history would be collected and a complete physical examination would be performed. This type of assessment is also called a **nursing database.**

Because it is thorough and complete, a comprehensive assessment can take a considerable amount of time and may require more than one client encounter to complete. For instance, an elderly client with a long history of emphysema is admitted to the hospital. Although the client is very cooperative during the admission history, the nurse notes that the client is becoming increasingly breathless. Using her clinical judgment, the nurse decides to defer completion of the nursing history until the client has had an opportunity to rest.

When a nurse performs a comprehensive assessment, it is to collect general information about the client, rather than specific information about an actual or possible problem. The purpose of a comprehensive assessment is to develop a database that suggests nursing diagnoses and collaborative problems. See Appendix B for a sample format of a comprehensive nursing history using a functional health pattern format. See Appendix C for a sample outline of a comprehensive physical examination.

Focused Assessment

A **focused assessment** involves the collection of information relevant to a specific problem identified by the client or suspected by the nurse as a result of a comprehensive or screening assessment. For instance, if a client identifies diarrhea as a problem during the comprehensive assessment, the nurse would collect specific subjective and objective data as outlined in Table 3-1. When the client reports that a particular symptom is present, the nurse must use a systematic approach in analyzing that symptom. Pain, dyspnea, fatigue, anxiety, and nausea are examples of symptoms that would need further investigation. Table 3-2 lists a method of investigating a symptom that includes the topic of the inquiry, sample questions, and how to record the response. Usually the nurse interrupts the flow of the interview to analyze a symptom at the time it is mentioned rather than waiting until the end of the formal interview.

In addition, the clustering of cues during data analysis may provide direction for a specific focused assessment generally associated with a particular nursing diagnosis. For example, if the clustering of cues suggests a nursing diagnosis of *impaired swallowing,* the nurse would use a focused assessment to gather additional subjective and objective data such as history of problem, weight change, coping pattern, height and weight, hydration status, neuromuscular status, and the presence of mechanical obstruction.

Screening Assessment

The final type of assessment a nurse might perform is a **screening assessment.** This is usually a brief assessment, limited in scope to a particular health problem such as glaucoma or hypertension, or to a specific body part such as the breasts or prostate gland. The purposes of a screening assessment include primary prevention (wellness promotion), case finding for secondary prevention, and ongoing surveillance.[16] Often the nurse will follow a protocol for screening assessments such as those recommended by the American Cancer Society related to screening for specific cancer sites (Table 3-3).

Ongoing Assessment

In addition to information collected during the different types of assessment, the nurse continues to collect data during each client contact. For example, on the

TABLE 3-1

Nursing Assessment of a Client with Diarrhea

Subjective Data

Important health information

Past health history: usual bowel habits, ingestion of coarse and spicy foods, recent travel, infections, stress, diverticulosis or malabsorption, metabolic disorders, inflammatory bowel disease, or irritable bowel syndrome

Medications: use of laxatives, magnesium-containing antacids, antibiotics, methyldopa, digitalis, colchicine, over-the-counter antidiarrheal medications

Functional health patterns

Nutritional/metabolic: weight loss, anorexia, thirst, borborygmi, bloating

Elimination: amount, frequency, color, character of stools

Activity/exercise: weakness

Cognitive/perceptual: tenesmus, abdominal pain and tenderness, cramping

Objective Data

General

Lethargy, sunken eyeballs, fever, malnutrition

Integumentary

Pallor, dry mucous membranes, poor skin turgor, perianal excoriation

Gastrointestinal

Amount, frequency, character (sudden onset, alternating diarrhea and constipation); color and consistency of stool; hyperactive bowel sounds; abdominal distention; presence of pus, blood, mucus, or fat in stools; fecal impaction

Urinary

Decreased output, concentrated urine

Possible findings

Abnormal serum electrolyte levels; anemia; leukocytosis; eosinophilia; positive stool cultures; presence of ova, parasites, leukocytes, blood, or fat in stools; abnormal sigmoidoscopic or colonoscopic findings; abnormal lower gastrointestinal series

From Lewis S, Collier I, Heitkemper M: *Medical-surgical nursing: assessment and management of clinical problems,* ed 4, St Louis, 1996, Mosby.

day following admission the client is seen in his hospital room, sleeping in bed, with intravenous fluids being administered and an indwelling catheter in place. The nurse now adds to the database in several patterns: nutrition pattern (intravenous fluids running), elimination pattern (indwelling catheter), and sleep/rest pattern (sleeping). In this and subsequent contacts with the client, the nurse will continue to collect data in all health patterns to keep interventions current and relevant. Questions to ask for each of the patterns are suggested in Appendix B.

T A B L E   3 - 2
Investigation of a Symptom

Location
Ask: "Where do you feel it? Where is it located?"
Record: Region of the body
         If local or radiating
         If superficial or deep

Quality
Ask: "What does it (feel, look) like?"
Record: The client's analogy (e.g., "Like being
         burned")

Quantity
Ask: "How often do you have this feeling? How
         bad is it? How much is it? How big is it?"
Record: Frequency (mild, moderate, severe), volume,
         size, extent, or number

Chronology
Ask: "When was the first time it occurred? Any
         particular time of day, week, month, or year?"
Record: Time of onset
         Duration
         Timing and frequency
         Course of symptoms

Setting
Ask: "Where are you when this occurs? What are
         you doing?"
Record: Where client is when the symptom occurs
         What client is doing
         If symptom is related to anything

Aggravating or Alleviating Factors
Ask: "What makes it better? Worse? Is there any
         activity that seems to cause it? What have you
         done for it? Did it help? Was there some
         reason you didn't do anything about it?"
Record: Influence of physical and emotional activities
         Client's attempts to alleviate (or treat)
         symptom

Associated Manifestations
Ask: "What other things do you see or feel when it
         occurs? Has it affected your appetite?
         Elimination? Sleeping?"
Record: Other symptoms

Meaning of the Symptom to the Patient
Ask: "How has it affected your life? Why have you
         sought care now? What do you think may be
         the cause?"
Record: Client's statements about effect of symptom
         and cause of symptom

From Lewis S, Collier I, Heitkemper M: *Medical-surgical nursing: assessment and management of clinical problems,* ed 4, St Louis, 1996, Mosby.

T A B L E   3 - 3
Examples of Screening for Specific Cancer Sites

SITE	SCREENING RECOMMENDATION
Skin	Self-examination monthly; physical examination every year; observation by client for sore that does not heal, change in wart or mole
Breast	Monthly breast self-examination; breast examination by health professional every 3 years for women ages 20 to 40 and every year after age 40; baseline mammogram at age 40, every 1 to 2 years between ages 40 and 49 (ask your doctor how often), and every year after age 50

From *Cancer facts and figures,* 1994, Atlanta, Ga, 1994, American Cancer Society.

Usually the nurse will collect data in all patterns of the functional health pattern framework. This is the preferred approach and should be used whenever possible. However, depending on the urgency of the situation or obviousness of the cue, the nurse may intervene for a problem/nursing diagnosis based on information from only one pattern. For example, if a client is having trouble clearing his airway because of thick, tenacious secretions, the nurse does not require further data to initiate interventions related to the nursing diagnosis of *impaired airway clearance* because of the life-threatening nature of this event.

Documentation

Once appropriate assessment data have been collected, it is necessary for the nurse to document data in the proper place. The specific format for documentation differs with the setting, but all formats serve the same purposes.

First, documenting the assessment findings provides a written, retrievable record on which to plan nursing care. If assessment data were not written, the amount, type, and quality of the information to be transmitted to other care providers would be neither systematic nor uniform. Although the amount of detail that is recorded may differ from nurse to nurse and involves a certain degree of judgment, most agencies have charting policies that help to standardize documentation.

Not only does written documentation aid in establishing an initial plan of care, it also helps in the evaluation process. By having written baseline data available for comparison, the nurse can monitor the effectiveness of planned interventions and adjust the plan as needed.

Documentation of assessment findings may also help to avoid repetition of time-consuming, tiring activities. For instance, if the nurse carefully documents the analysis of a client's hip pain, it is not necessary for other providers, such as a physical therapist, to obtain and document the same information. In addition to saving the professional's time, it also increases the client's confidence in the care providers by avoiding repetitious questioning that often leaves the client feeling as if nobody is really listening.

Careful documentation of assessment findings can also serve as a means of communicating important information to others in the same or different disciplines. For instance, the more functional approach of the nursing history may provide valuable insight to the client's physician, who is primarily interested in specific physiologic parameters.

Many nurse practice acts and practice standards mandate that assessment findings be documented. For instance, the Standards of Nursing Practice developed by the American Nurses' Association state:

STANDARD ONE
The collection of data about the health status of the client is systematic and continuous. These data are communicated to appropriate persons, recorded and stored in a retrievable and accessible system.[18]

Clearly, this statement leaves no doubt as to the professional responsibility all nurses share regarding documentation.

Another compelling reason to carefully record assessment findings relates to the need for a legal reference that is admissible in a court of law if questions arise related to care. The litigious nature of society today makes it imperative that nurses document their actions in a legally acceptable way to protect themselves in the event of a lawsuit. The truism, "If it's not written down, it was not done," reminds the practitioner of the personal and professional importance of documenting nursing actions.

Clustering Assessment Cues

As the nurse collects the assessment data, the data should be organized in a way that facilitates analysis (that is, using the functional health pattern framework) and leads to the identification of nursing diagnoses. Data are analyzed for their clarity, relevance, and validity. As this analysis proceeds, the nurse clusters related diagnostic cues.

TABLE 3-4
Analysis of Data
• Cue clarification
• Evaluation
• Reliability
• Validation

Data Analysis

It is critical that nursing diagnoses be supported by assessment data. The nurse should not assign a nursing diagnosis to a client situation without data to support it. The process of thinking about the data is called **analysis.**

As stated earlier, a cue is a clinically useful fact about the client's status. In analyzing the data, the nurse considers several questions related to the quality of the cues (Table 3-4).

1. Are there cues that need to be clarified? **Cue clarification** is the process of defining or explaining what the client means by the cue. For example, a client may state that he understands his medical diagnosis. It is not uncommon to have clients say they "understand" only to have further questioning uncover large gaps in their knowledge. Having the client explain what he means by "I understand" clarifies exactly what the client knows.

2. Does the nurse need more information in order to evaluate the data? **Evaluation** of the data occurs as the nurse estimates the importance and completeness of the cues. In order to make this evaluation, the nurse uses knowledge and experience to critically analyze the data. For example, a client may say his appetite has decreased. This may or may not be an important cue. Other information that the nurse needs in order to evaluate the client's reported decrease in appetite could include:
   • when this change was first noted
   • any weight change
   • any emotional problems that may be affecting the client's appetite
   • any explanations from the client to account for this change.

3. Are the data reliable? **Reliability** refers to the amount of confidence the nurse has in the trustworthiness of the data. The nurse first judges the

reliability of the person giving the information. The nurse can determine this in part based on the person's assessed physical and mental status. In evaluating reliability the nurse also looks for incongruencies among various sources of information. For example, a client may state she is 76, but her chart lists her age as 83. These two pieces of data are incongruent and therefore one or both may be unreliable. Reliability of data is also based on the nurse's judgment. Do the data make sense or do they seem illogical? Recall that in critical thinking it is important to keep an open mind; however, the nurse must still apply common sense.

4. Have the data been validated? **Validation** is the process of confirming or substantiating the data. Methods of validation include directly observing the cue, rechecking your own data, eliciting the help of a colleague in examining the data, and considering the congruency of what the nurse has observed and what the client has stated.[18]

The very important step of analyzing data by using one or more of these acts—clarifying, evaluating, determining reliability, and validating—is critical to the nurse's thinking process about the data. Accurate analysis of the data helps to prevent mistakes that could result in diagnostic error.

Data/Cue Clustering

When the nurse is satisfied that sufficient data have been collected to warrant further analysis, the process of clustering can begin. **Clustering** is the grouping of data into logically associated units of information. Clustering the data into useful units results in a smaller, more manageable number of units. This simplifies the task of analysis.

There are several ways to cluster data. Initially the data should be organized into appropriate functional health patterns. In order to do this the nurse needs to have a clear understanding of what types of data are included in each functional health pattern. Study of the topics included in each pattern familiarizes the nurse with the types of information pertinent to each pattern (see Appendix A). When all the data have been clustered in this manner, it is easier to identify functional and dysfunctional patterns.

The following example demonstrates clustering of data for Ms. Smith into functional health patterns.

Health Perception/Health Management Pattern

1. Doesn't get annual physical exams
2. Doesn't exercise, rarely ill

3. Takes over-the-counter aspirin for control of pain caused by arthritis.

Nutritional/Metabolic Pattern

1. Twenty-pound weight gain over the past year
2. Does not know the recommended foods from the "Food Pyramid"
3. Frequently does not eat breakfast and often eats a high fat diet
4. 5′4″; 145 pounds
5. Appears moderately obese with intact skin
6. Hair shiny and well kept

Elimination Pattern

1. Voids about every four hours, urine clear and pale yellow
2. Bowel movements every two to three days, firm and brown

Activity/Exercise Pattern

1. Low energy; able to perform all activities of daily living
2. Works a 60-hour week and rarely has any leisure activity
3. Vital signs are 134/90; 84; 22; T98.6

Cognitive/Perceptual pattern

1. Wears glasses, hears whispered words at two feet
2. Denies pain other than occasional headache
3. Learns easily when explanation given

Sleep/Rest Pattern

1. Often tired during the day
2. Does not usually nap; hour of sleep 9 P.M.
3. Frequent awakenings during the night
4. Often awakens in the early morning and is unable to return to sleep
5. Usually gets up at 5:30 A.M., appears tired with dark circles under eyes; alert

Self-Perception/Self-Concept Pattern

1. Expresses dissatisfaction with weight gain
2. Feels overworked and undervalued by her employer and her husband
3. Expresses pride in her work
4. Articulate and sociable

Role/Relationship Pattern

1. Husband out of work
2. Husband began using drugs and alcohol again
3. Cried when talking about this
4. States has frequent fights with husband
5. Described some work stress but has good relationships with several of her co-workers

Sexuality/Reproductive Pattern

1. Has not had sexual relations with husband in more than six months
2. Has no children and does not plan children at this time
3. Expressed dissatisfaction about her sexual relationship with husband

Coping/Stress Tolerance Pattern

1. Tries to discuss her work and her frustrations about husband's drinking and unemployment with him
2. Admits to getting very angry and swearing and shouting
3. Denies any physical abuse
4. Finds that she eats greater quantities and more often to make herself feel better
5. Denies regular exercise
6. Bears most of the discomfort of her life alone; occasionally talks with co-workers but does not discuss these issues with family; appears tired, listless

Value/Belief Pattern

1. Rarely goes to church anymore as husband does not want to go
2. Misses this in her life

When the nurse uses only this framework to cluster the data, nursing diagnoses are made solely on the basis of data clustered within one pattern. For example, the following nursing diagnoses are made for Ms. Smith from the respective functional health patterns:

Health perception/health management pattern: *altered health maintenance related to failure to obtain preventive health care*

Nutritional/metabolic pattern: *altered nutrition: more than body requirements related to caloric intake greater than energy expenditure*

Sleep/rest pattern: *sleep pattern disturbance related to unknown etiology.*

Reclustering

This method would continue for all of the functional health patterns. Although accurate diagnoses can often be made by this method, the related factors may be unclear or incomplete when based only on data from one pattern. A better way to cluster data is to add a second step to the process of clustering before making any nursing diagnosis.

This second step is to **recluster** data based on the general problem areas that can be identified from the initial clustering. Reclustering involves grouping related data from the different patterns. For example, based on the case presented, the nurse would identify

---

TABLE 3-5

Identifying a Dysfunctional Pattern

- Note a change from the client's usual pattern
- Note a deviation from normal parameters for a given age-group, sex, or developmental stage

---

a general problem area of weight gain based on dysfunction in the nutritional/metabolic pattern and look for other related cues from all of the functional health patterns.

Differentiation between functional and dysfunctional patterns assists in identifying general problem areas. This process begins by noting a **change** in the client's status (for example, 20 pound weight gain) or a **deviation** from the expected norm (such as awakening frequently at night) (Table 3-5).

From the data given in the example for Ms. Smith, clinically relevant cues have been reclustered together in order to make a nursing diagnosis.

General problem area: weight gain
Reclustered Data:
- Twenty-pound weight gain
- 5′4″, 145 pounds
- No breakfast
- High-fat foods
- Minimal nutrition knowledge
- No exercise
- Eats to feel better

Nursing Diagnosis:
Altered nutrition: more than body requirements related to lack of knowledge of proper diet, stress-related eating, and inadequate exercise as manifested by being more than 20% above ideal body weight

This method results in a more accurate diagnosis since it is based on clustering data from different patterns together. Analysis of the reclustered data makes the nursing diagnosis obvious to the nurse (for instance, *altered nutrition: more than body requirements)* and the related factors of the problem are identifiable from data in the other patterns. Note how much more specific the related to statement is than when the same diagnosis was made based on data from the nutritional/metabolic pattern alone. This specificity is important in guiding nursing interventions. This method of clustering and reclustering is used throughout the case studies in this text.

Clustering also occurs based on the nurse's past experience. Through experience the nurse learns that certain cues "go together." Take, for example, the occurrence of prolonged immobility in an elderly client with urinary incontinence. The nurse clusters these cues together and identifies the nursing diagnosis of *risk for impaired skin integrity* based on experience.

Another way clustering may occur is when a nursing diagnosis is immediately suggested to the nurse by a single cue (for example, sores on the client's tongue and gums). To strengthen the diagnostic accuracy, the nurse looks for additional supporting data from within the database that would support the nursing diagnosis of *altered oral mucous membrane*. Since the sores represent the major defining characteristics for this diagnosis, the nurse would assess the client for the presence of additional major and minor defining characteristics including coating on the tongue, dry mouth, and edema. The presence of the major defining characteristic, the critical indicator of a nursing diagnosis, always offers strong support for the nursing diagnosis. Thus the major defining characteristic is considered a highly relevant cue. As the novice nurse begins to learn the major defining characteristics associated with each diagnosis, it becomes easier to connect relevant cues with the correct nursing diagnosis.

When a diagnostically relevant cue is present but there are no other data available to support a nursing diagnosis, the nurse may perform a focused assessment to collect more data in order to "rule in" or "rule out" a nursing diagnosis. The following example illustrates this process.

Mrs. Rankin is a 73-year-old woman who comes to your clinic because of a long history of insomnia. Based on a diagnostically relevant cue of insomnia, you perform a focused assessment related to her sleep history. The client states that she goes to bed around 8:00 P.M. nightly and falls asleep in about one hour. She usually sleeps soundly for about four or five hours, awakens, and cannot fall back to sleep. She stays in bed, hoping that sleep will return. She finally gets out of bed around 5:30 A.M., feeling tired and sluggish. She states that she dozes frequently during the day. Her bedtime ritual includes drinking a cup of hot coffee with cream and sugar. She has dark circles under her eyes. She "nods off" occasionally during the interview process.

The nurse recognizes many cues here that fit into the sleep/rest pattern. This is the pattern that describes patterns of sleep, rest, and relaxation. In this instance, cues cluster easily from this one pattern. Analysis of the cues suggests a possible cause for the sleep problem—drinking coffee before bedtime.

Once the related cues have been clustered from within the pattern and reclustered from across different patterns, it becomes easier to determine whether or not there is a problem. Some of the cues and patterns may not be dysfunctional but rather may reflect strengths of the client. The nurse needs to remember to consider these strengths in planning the client's care. For example, in the earlier client scenario, Ms. Smith reported good relationships with her co-workers. This is a strength that could be used by the nurse to suggest an "exercise buddy" from work for a noontime walk.

These are some of the possible ways for data to be linked together. Using a complete database is important when clustering because the nurse needs to consider data from all the client's patterns. This holistic view of the individual adds significantly more data, which enables the nurse to make nursing diagnoses based on a complete picture of the individual.

Once the nurse has grouped relevant cues into clusters and made some initial inferences about their meaning, the process of developing a nursing diagnosis can proceed. According to the diagnostic process model (see Fig. 3-1), the next steps include the proposal of diagnostic hypotheses, the testing of hypotheses, and the selection of an accurate diagnosis.

Proposing Diagnostic Hypotheses

The process of making a nursing diagnosis from clustered cues begins with the recognition of general client problems or issues. These general problems are useful in guiding the collection of additional assessment data and providing direction in selecting possible nursing diagnoses. But general ideas about client problems are not specific enough to be useful in planning individualized care. In making a diagnosis, the nurse must refine thinking about general problems by using a reasoning process. As a part of this process the nurse recalls knowledge of specific nursing diagnoses. The nurse compares knowledge about various diagnoses to the data collected and the general problems identified for an individual client. Next, the nurse proposes several likely diagnostic explanations for the findings. These tentative nursing diagnoses are called **diagnostic hypotheses** because they represent the nurse's prediction of what the most correct nursing diagnosis might be. In some instances cues exist that so clearly support a single nursing diagnosis that it is unnecessary to consider alternative diagnostic hypotheses. However, this situation is the exception and not the rule. It is usually necessary to consider more than one diagnostic hypothesis before selecting the most accurate diagnosis.

Consider this example: You are performing an assessment on Gina, a 17-year-old female who is reported to be having some difficulty in school. You collect the following information:

- Teachers have complained about Gina's restlessness, incomplete work, and decline in performance.
- She has weight loss of 16 pounds in the last eight weeks. Her current weight is 102 pounds; she is 5'6" tall.
- Gina's mother expresses concern over Gina's "poor eating habits." Gina herself is not concerned about her weight loss but complains of feeling moody, irritable, and jumpy. She is also having difficulty sleeping. She states that her appetite is huge and she is not dieting.

From this initial data, some general problem areas come to mind. These include:

1. Nutrition problem
2. Sleep problem
3. Change in school performance and temperament

The exact alterations are not yet clear. The initial clusters of information are enough to lead the nurse to perform a more extensive assessment focused on the nutritional/metabolic, sleep/rest, and cognitive/perceptual patterns. Until additional data are collected and analyzed, it is not possible to assign a specific name (diagnosis) to this client's problem or to plan care.

Let's look more closely at just one of the areas of concern: the nutrition problem. Some of the additional data that the nurse would collect include specific eating habits of concern to the mother, the quantity and types of food Gina is eating, and Gina's basic understanding of nutrition.

The nurse might also explore whether this client has other signs and symptoms of metabolic disorders that occur in this age-group. For example, does she have polyuria or excessive thirst? Does she have an elevated heart rate or exophthalmos? This requires a reexamination of all the functional health patterns to identify and recluster the data. While the nurse is not responsible for diagnosing a metabolic disorder such as diabetes or hyperthyroidism, the nurse should collect related data based on her knowledge of pathophysiology and disease processes. These data can then be used by other health care providers in making a medical diagnosis and can be used by the nurse in identifying collaborative problems. The client's responses to newly diagnosed diseases may also lead to the identification of nursing diagnoses.

In this case, further assessment of the nutrition/metabolic pattern, including a diet recall, showed that Gina was consuming more than the expected amount of calories for her age, weight, and exercise level. She consumed a large amount of high-calorie, low-nutrition snack food and was unable to describe more nutritious food choices. She also showed signs of increased metabolic rate (elevated heart rate, restlessness, flushed skin, weight loss despite large caloric intake). Based on these data two very different diagnostic hypotheses related to nutritional status could be considered for this client. The first is *altered nutrition: more than body requirements related to lack of knowledge of low-calorie, high-nutrition foods as evidenced by client report of large intake of high-calorie snacks and inability to name nutritious alternatives.* The second diagnostic hypothesis that may be considered for this client is *altered nutrition: less than body requirements related to increased caloric needs secondary to elevated metabolic rate.*

At this point in the diagnostic process the nurse has moved from a general problem to the proposal of two specific diagnostic hypotheses. The next step will be to examine each hypothesis and select the more accurate of the two.

With experience it becomes easier to generate diagnostic hypotheses. An expert nurse has a fund of experience from which to draw. This allows the nurse to recognize that in the past, clients with similar findings had certain nursing diagnoses. The nurse learns to recognize assessment data that support these diagnoses. This leads to an integration of clinical knowledge, experience, and diagnostic expertise in the experienced clinician.

The student or novice nurse does not have this broad base of experience to help in making a nursing diagnosis. The student/novice is often confronted with entirely new client problems and diagnoses outside the scope of experience. How can the student/novice build the diagnostic skills needed in practice? There are a number of tools that the beginner can use to generate diagnostic hypotheses. These tools include lists of nursing diagnoses associated with problems in each functional health pattern (see Appendix D). Such a list can help structure thinking about possible diagnoses for which the nurse has incomplete knowledge or limited experience. A complete reference that contains each nursing diagnosis along with its definition and defining characteristics is an essential tool. These references help link significant assessment findings with nursing diagnoses and are a tremendous aid in acquiring diagnostic skills. Collaboration and consultation with expert nurses are also invaluable aids in refining diagnostic reasoning skills. The beginning nurse must use a variety of resources plus a conscious thought process to make sense of the data collected and to generate possible diagnostic explanations.

Testing Diagnostic Hypotheses

Once the nurse has generated a list of the most likely nursing diagnoses (diagnostic hypotheses) a decision must be made as to which diagnosis best represents the client problem. This occurs through hypothesis testing. **Hypothesis testing** is a process in which each diagnostic hypothesis is evaluated. As a result of this evaluation inaccurate diagnoses are eliminated and an accurate diagnosis is selected.

Choosing the most accurate diagnosis is not always an easy task. The diagnostic labels, which are the official "names" of the nursing diagnoses, do not contain information on the meaning of the diagnoses. It is difficult to distinguish between similar diagnoses without additional information about the meaning, or definition, of the diagnostic labels. For example, *fear* and *anxiety* are both nursing diagnoses. Although they have some common threads, they are not synonymous. The nurse must become familiar with the definitions of diagnoses in order to accurately apply them to specific client situations.

In addition to the definition, the defining characteristics of a diagnostic label also guide the use of that diagnosis. In the process of hypothesis testing, the nurse must decide which proposed diagnosis is most consistent with the assessment cues. Knowing the defining characteristics for all diagnoses under consideration helps guide the collection of additional focused assessment data. These data are then compared to the defining characteristics of each diagnostic hypothesis to identify the accuracy of the diagnostic alternatives.

In the earlier example, two diagnostic hypotheses were considered for 17-year-old Gina. The first was *altered nutrition: more than body requirements related to lack of knowledge of low-calorie, high-nutrition foods.* Two cues are present to support this diagnosis: her reported intake of "junk" food and her inadequate knowledge of healthier food choices. However, the major defining characteristic for the diagnosis *altered nutrition: more than body requirements* is the finding that the client is overweight or obese. Another defining characteristic is that the client consumes calories in excess of her metabolic needs. This is clearly not true of this particular client who has lost weight over the previous eight weeks. She does not fit the definition of this diagnosis even though she does have excessive intake of some snack foods and a high calorie intake. Through the process of hypothesis testing this diagnosis can be eliminated from consideration.

The second diagnostic hypothesis in this case was *altered nutrition: less than body requirements related to increased caloric needs secondary to elevated meta-bolic rate.* Several cues support this diagnosis, including weight loss, weight below ideal for height, and additional signs of increased metabolic rate including restlessness, irritability, and increased heart rate. There are no conflicting cues that would eliminate this diagnosis. The process of hypothesis testing confirms that this is an accurate nursing diagnosis. In addition to this nursing diagnosis, the medical diagnosis of hyperthyroidism was made by the physician. As part of Gina's ongoing care the physician will focus on treating the hyperthyroidism. Nursing care will focus on helping Gina to meet her increased caloric needs in a nutritious fashion and preventing further weight loss.

Selecting an Accurate Diagnosis

The diagnostic process results in the identification of the most accurate nursing diagnosis based on individual client data. In the above example, two diagnoses were considered and the selection of the most accurate diagnosis was made by comparing the existing assessment data to the definition and defining characteristics for each diagnosis. In clinical practice, decision making is often more complex. The nurse may have to discriminate between multiple diagnostic possibilities, several of which are consistent with some of the cues present. Consider the following case:

Mr. Andrews is a 38-year-old married man with four children. His father recently died from Huntington's disease. His grandfather also died from this disease. Mr. Andrews reports that he is considering undergoing the genetic test that will tell him if he too will develop this devastating illness. He is unsure if he really wants to have this information. He tells you that he would like to know if he does *not* carry the gene for Huntington's disease. He would especially like to know if his children are at risk or not. (If Mr. Andrews has the gene for Huntington's, he will develop the disease; his children will each have a 50% chance of developing the disease. If he does not carry the gene, neither he nor his children are at risk. Huntington's disease strikes in the middle adult years and is a fatal, degenerative, neurologic disorder.) On the other hand, he would prefer not to know if he does carry the gene for this disease. He is not sure how he would handle knowing he would certainly die from Huntington's. He is now healthy and without symptoms. He states, "Maybe it would help me plan if I did know I would have a short life." He states he is afraid to die in the way his father and grandfather did. He is unable to decide.

As Mr. Andrews' nurse, you consider the following list of diagnostic alternatives:

1. *Fear related to dying of Huntington's disease*
2. *Anxiety related to possibly having Huntington's disease*
3. *Decisional conflict related to advantages and disadvantages to self and children of knowing results of genetic screening for Huntington's disease.*

In this situation, data exist to support more than one of these diagnoses. The nurse must determine which diagnoses most accurately reflect the client's problems and are most useful in planning nursing care. Consider each diagnosis: Mr. Andrews is clearly afraid of developing this disease. He has expressed this fear verbally. The definition of *fear* is "a feeling of dread related to an identifiable source which the person validates."[3] The client's ability to identify the source or object of the fear is the defining characteristic of this diagnosis. This client's behavior is consistent with both the definition and defining characteristics of *fear* and so this remains a viable diagnostic possibility. *Anxiety* can be ruled out as a diagnosis. There is a clear focus to this client's discomfort, which is inconsistent with the definition for the diagnosis *anxiety* ("a vague uneasy feeling whose source is nonspecific or unknown to the individual"[3]). Mr. Andrews is having difficulty making a decision about whether or not to undergo genetic testing. This decision is very important to him; he is taking a risk no matter which decision he makes. The nursing diagnosis *decisional conflict* is defined as "the state of uncertainty about course of action to be taken when choice among competing actions involves risk, loss, or challenge to personal life values."[3] Mr. Andrews' responses are consistent with this definition.

At this point in the diagnostic process, the nurse must decide which diagnosis is most accurate. While fear is an issue for this client, he is not seeking help for dealing with his fear at this point. He knows that he may or may not have something to fear, as his chance of inheriting this disease from his father is 50%. He may have the disease he may not. The issue of immediate concern to Mr. Andrews is his desire to make a decision regarding genetic testing. He has conflicting needs and desires surrounding this issue. He has verbalized his uncertainty about the choices and the disadvantages of testing or not testing. He is examining his own values about knowing he is disease free or knowing he will develop this disease. These findings are the defining characteristics for the diagnosis *decisional conflict*. A clear cluster of cues supports this nursing diagnosis. *Decisional conflict* is the most accurate and clinically useful diagnosis for this client at this time. This diagnosis can be validated by discussing it with the client. Once validated, the nurse works with the client to develop expected outcomes. For example, an expected outcome for this client might be that the client will make a decision regarding genetic testing by his next visit. Interventions are then designed to help the client achieve the goals (such as, introduce client to a resource person from the Huntington's disease support group; discuss the advantages and disadvantages of early knowledge regarding Huntington's disease; suggest talking to a geneticist about accuracy of testing; suggest consultation with religious advisor). The evaluation process will examine whether or not the client has been able to make a decision regarding genetic testing.

The process of making a nursing diagnosis includes the development of several alternative diagnostic hypotheses. These diagnostic possibilities are derived from the data that are collected and organized during assessment. Diagnostic hypotheses are predictions about which diagnostic labels may most accurately describe the client's problem. Each alternative diagnosis is confirmed or ruled out by comparing the definition and defining characteristics of the diagnosis with the assessment data. The most accurate diagnosis is selected and used as the basis for planning care.

Minimizing Sources of Diagnostic Errors

The ability to write accurate nursing diagnoses is a learned skill. As with any new skill, the learner can expect frustration and annoyance on the way to competence. The student can expect to make many diagnostic errors along the way, but persistence has its own reward!

Lunney offers some comfort to the neophyte nursing diagnostician when she states that the accuracy of a nursing diagnosis should not be considered a dichotomous variable.[4] In other words, a nursing diagnosis is neither totally "accurate" nor totally "inaccurate." Rather, accuracy can be thought of as a matter of degree. Table 3-6 describes a seven-point scale of accuracy developed by Lunney, with criteria for each point on the scale.[4] With increased knowledge, experience, practice, and supervision, the learner can move up the scale of accuracy. As the nurse becomes more accurate at making nursing diagnoses, satisfaction with this phase of professional practice will increase.

Although nurse satisfaction is one important reason for making accurate nursing diagnoses, the most important reasons are client-based. First, a nursing diagnosis could be made where none exists. The resulting unnecessary interventions could confuse the client, lessen confidence in the nurse, and actually cause

TABLE 3-6	
Ordinal Scale for Degrees of Accuracy*	
VALUE	**CRITERIA**
+5	Diagnosis is consistent with all of the cues, supported by highly relevant cues, and precise
+4	Diagnosis is consistent with most or all of the cues and supported by relevant cues but fails to reflect one or a few highly relevant cues
+3	Diagnosis is consistent with many of the cues but fails to reflect the specificity of available cues
+2	Diagnosis is indicated by some of the cues but there are insufficient cues relevant to the diagnosis and/or the diagnosis is a lower priority than other diagnoses
+1	Diagnosis is only suggested by one or a few cues
0	Diagnosis is not indicated by any of the cues; no diagnosis is stated when there are sufficient cues to state a diagnosis; the diagnosis cannot be rated
−1	Diagnosis is indicated by more than one cue but should be rejected based on the presence of at least two disconfirming cues

From Lunney M: Accuracy of nursing diagnoses: concept development, *Nursing Diagnosis* 1:16, 1990.
*Higher positive number indicates greater accuracy.

TABLE 3-7
Sources of Diagnostic Error
Collecting
Insufficient data
Too much data
Lack of knowledge/skill
Failure to generate multiple hypotheses
Interpreting
Inaccurate interpretation of cues
Failure to consider conflicting cues
Using an insufficient number of cues
Using unreliable or invalid data
Failure to consider cultural influences or developmental stage
Clustering
Insufficient cluster of cues
Premature or early closure
Incorrect clustering
Labeling
Wrong diagnostic label selected
Condition is a collaborative problem
Failure to validate nursing diagnosis with patient
Failure to seek guidance

harm. Or, a nursing diagnosis might not be identified when one does exist. This results in failure to treat and could cause serious delay in treatment or harm to the client. An inaccurately written diagnosis could likewise cause delay in initiating appropriate treatment as well as cause harm to the client.

A discussion of some of the sources of diagnostic error is beneficial to the learner. Awareness of sources of error can alert the nurse to areas that need special attention and increase accuracy. Gordon uses four categories to look at sources of diagnostic error—collecting, interpreting, clustering, and labeling.[2] Table 3-7 summarizes the sources of diagnostic error.

Errors in Collecting
Insufficient Data
When insufficient data are collected, the nurse may fail to see that a problem exists. For example, if the nurse does not complete an adequate dietary history, the nurse may fail to identify a problem from the nutritional/metabolic pattern such as *risk for altered nutrition: more than body requirements*.

To avoid this source of error, the nurse needs to assess the client in all functional health patterns. If a problem is noted in a particular pattern, a focused assessment of that pattern and related patterns is indicated.

Too Much Data
It is possible for the nurse to collect or have available too much information. If this large amount of information is disorganized, it will further confuse the attempt to identify client problems. Often when dealing with a large amount of information, much of that information is irrelevant. When large amounts of irrelevant data are available, they can lead to confusion and inertia. Consider the client admitted to the hospital for the third time in two weeks. Information available to the nurse might include previous hospital records, a report from the home health nurse, a social service report, the ambulance report, admission x-rays and lab values, and the admission history and physical done by the intern. Add to this the information that the client and his daughter are anxious to recount, and you have a potentially overwhelming situation.

To avoid diagnostic error caused by too much information, the nurse can do several things. First, the nurse needs to make a judgment about the best source for information necessary to meet the client's most urgent needs. The nurse may decide to complete a nursing history (still more data!) to determine the client's response to his health status. If the situation is more urgent, the nurse may use the intern's history and physical examination, and the ambulance report. Once an initial plan is in place, the nurse can then decide what information might add additional insight into the plan of care for the client.

Lack of Knowledge and Skill

Inadequate knowledge and skill to perform necessary assessments may hamper the nurse in collecting the critical signs and symptoms associated with a particular nursing diagnosis. For instance, difficulty with communication skills could make it hard for the nurse to gather the subjective information from the client to support the nursing diagnosis of *hopelessness*. Or, lack of knowledge in interpreting arterial blood gases might cause the nurse to miss the nursing diagnosis of *dysfunctional ventilatory weaning response: severe.*

The obvious way to eliminate lack of knowledge and skill as a source of diagnostic error is to broaden and deepen one's clinical knowledge base. However, cognitive and psychomotor skills are learned over time, and based on formal learning and practice. If the nurse recognizes that lack of knowledge and skill may be a factor, it is imperative that a more experienced nurse be consulted to avoid a potentially serious error. The nurse can benefit from this interaction and can be assured that knowledge and skill level will increase with experience and study.

Failure to Generate Multiple Hypotheses

Although failure to generate multiple hypotheses is a potential source of error in interpreting data, it is also a source of error in collecting data as well. When the nurse fails to generate multiple hypotheses, important assessment information that could confirm or refute potential diagnoses is not collected. Usually the experienced nurse is considering multiple diagnostic hypotheses concurrently with data collection. These possible hypotheses direct the nurse to do branching questioning and assessing to determine the presence of critical defining characteristics.

For example, the nurse may quickly diagnose a client's complaint of lack of energy as *fatigue*. Because the nurse only generated one hypothesis, insufficient data were gathered on other possibly relevant diagnoses such as *activity intolerance* or *sleep pattern disturbance*. Additional assessments such as physiologic responses to activity and a sleep history would have been performed had other diagnostic hypotheses been considered. This additional consideration would have made the most accurate diagnosis more readily apparent.

Errors in Interpreting Data
Inaccurate Interpretation of Cues

Once data have been collected the nurse reviews the information with the idea of interpreting the data. At this point in the diagnostic process, errors can be made in two ways. First, the nurse can make an error of omission by not recognizing that a cue is a major or minor defining characteristic of a specific diagnosis. Or, the nurse can make an error of commission, assigning a diagnosis to a cue that is not relevant to the diagnosis. This type of error is most often made by the nurse who is clinically inexperienced or new to nursing diagnosis. Generally these types of errors will diminish as the nurse gains experience and knowledge in nursing diagnosis. Use of nursing diagnosis reference books helps to prevent this type of error.

Failure to Consider Conflicting Cues

In some instances the nurse may recognize that a cue or set of cues is associated with a nursing diagnosis. The nurse may fail, however, to consider conflicting or disconfirming cues. **Conflicting cues** are items of information that may negate the validity of a particular nursing diagnosis. For instance, a client presents with the following signs and symptoms: weight gain of 15 pounds in past three weeks, peripheral edema, and taut shiny skin of the lower extremities. The nurse makes the diagnosis of *altered nutrition: more than body requirements* because the weight gain made the person 14% over ideal weight, a major defining characteristic for this diagnosis. The nurse failed to consider the conflicting cues of edema and taut shiny skin, which suggest a diagnosis of *fluid volume excess*. These cues negate the diagnosis of *altered nutrition: more than body requirements*.

Using an Insufficient Number of Cues

It is important that the nurse base a nursing diagnosis on a sufficient number of valid cues to ensure the accuracy of the diagnosis. There are some instances where a single cue is so indicative of a diagnosis that it is sufficient to attach the label. For instance, the client's expressed desire to seek information for the purpose of health promotion is sufficient to assign the diagnosis of *health-seeking behavior*. In most instances, however, it is a much better practice to identify a group of cues specific to a diagnosis. This helps to ensure accuracy. If a sufficient number of cues are not available or the nurse is uncomfortable with the diagnosis, the collection of additional data can help clarify the issue.

A similar mistake can occur when looking at cues in isolation rather than in the context of the entire client situation. For instance, when a client refuses to take a medication, the nurse may prematurely assign the diagnosis of *noncompliance*. The collection of additional data would help the nurse decide if *noncompliance* is an accurate diagnosis or not. For example, if the nurse learns that the drug caused the client to have severe diarrhea, then *noncompliance* is not an appropriate diagnosis.

Using Unreliable or Invalid Data

When the data used to support a diagnosis are unreliable or invalid, the resulting diagnosis could be in error. Unreliable data can result from many causes, such as a cognitive impairment or intoxication of the client or faulty instrumentation. If cognitive impairment is present, for instance, subjective information provided by the client could be invalid. The client might deny a problem with urinary incontinence when in fact it has been a problem for some time. Or, if faulty instrumentation is a problem, the sphygmomanometer could give a blood pressure reading of 140/90 when the blood pressure was actually 80/50.

The nurse should be suspicious of incongruity in a client's story or in the facts presented by a knowledgeable other. If the information presented seems to be unreliable, the nurse must seek validation before these data can be used as cues to a diagnosis.

Failure to Consider Cultural Influence or Developmental Stage

It is important that the nurse be culturally sensitive in interpreting cues. When the nurse is not certain of the meaning of a cue, it is important to ask the client for interpretation. For instance, in some cultures it is desirable for the women to be full-figured. To assign the diagnosis of *altered nutrition: more than body requirements* to a woman who held this belief could constitute an error in diagnosis.

Failure to consider the client's developmental stage can also influence the interpretation of data and lead to a diagnostic error. For instance, one of the tasks of the older adult is body transcendence versus body preoccupation.[19] This involves recognizing physical decline but rising above aches and pains so that happiness is not defined by physical well-being. If the client has accomplished this task, she may not be a candidate for the diagnosis of *self-concept disturbance related to graying hair*.

Errors in Clustering
Insufficient Cluster of Cues

When the cluster of cues is insufficient to warrant a specific diagnosis, the nurse should avoid the temptation to "fudge" and assign the diagnosis anyway. Instead, the nurse might designate the diagnosis as a "possible." If the clustering is inadequate or vague, the nurse may be unable to assign a diagnosis until the client's situation develops further or additional data can be collected.

Premature or Early Closure

The nurse may make a diagnostic judgment too early to ensure accuracy. For instance, the nurse may decide on a nursing diagnosis before the nursing history has been completed, pertinent lab work is available, or the client's family can be interviewed. Although the cues were clustered appropriately, the nurse was too hasty and may have jumped to an erroneous conclusion by not considering or collecting all pertinent data.

Incorrect Clustering of Cues

If the nurse clusters cues incorrectly, it could lead to an error in diagnosis. Generally, this error is based on an inadequate knowledge base and lack of familiarity with related cues. A good solution to this problem is for the nurse to have a current nursing diagnosis book available for easy reference. According to Gordon, "Lack of standardization of diagnostic categories used in nursing diagnosis contributes to this type of error."[2] Because the widespread use of nursing diagnosis is relatively new, the nurse is cautioned to use accepted signs, symptoms, and category definitions when writing diagnoses.

Errors in Labeling
Wrong Diagnostic Label Selected

This situation is an obvious error on the part of the nurse. The wrong diagnosis has been selected. Some part of the process of making a diagnostic judgment was omitted or done incorrectly, and an inaccurate diagnosis resulted. Often the cause of this error is lack of knowledge on the part of the nurse or insufficient cues or data collection. Because the diagnostic label directs subsequent nursing interventions, there is an inherent danger in this error. If the diagnosis is incorrect, the interventions could also be incorrect and potentially harmful to the client. Also, because the wrong diagnosis was made, the correct diagnosis and subsequent nursing interventions are not part of the plan. The way to avoid this error is to perform each step of the diagnostic reasoning process carefully and thoughtfully, making certain that sufficient cues are available. The inexperienced nurse would do well to have an experienced co-worker validate the accuracy of the diagnosis.

Failure to Validate Nursing Diagnosis with Client

Diagnostic reasoning and nursing diagnosis involve complex reasoning. Because of this complexity, the nurse often excludes the client from the deliberations around this process. However, failure to validate the nursing diagnosis with the client could lead to serious diagnostic error. The client can be given a clear explanation of what the nurse identifies as the major problem or problems that need interventions. Not only will client validation increase accuracy, it will also help the client to become a contributing member of the team dedicated to his care.

Condition is a Collaborative Problem

Collaborative problems, written as *potential complication,* have been discussed previously. Often, the nurse has difficulty differentiating a collaborative problem from a nursing diagnosis. For instance, would the nurse select *PC: increased intracranial pressure* (potential complication) or *altered thought processes* (nursing diagnosis) for a cluster of cues that included inaccurate interpretation of surroundings, disorientation, metastatic brain tumor, and decrease in motor function? In this case, although there are important interventions from both disciplines, the primary treatment for the problem is clearly in the realm of medicine. The nurse should judge this to be a collaborative problem and would write *PC: increased intracranial pressure.*

Failure to Seek Guidance

A very common source of error for the nurse inexperienced in the diagnostic reasoning process is failure to seek guidance when needed. Nursing faculty and experienced clinicians are available resources to the student. The experienced nurse can be consulted at any point in the process for direction. Once the diagnosis has been developed, it is good practice to validate it with a knowledgeable person. Even if advice is not sought earlier in the process, it is strongly recommended that the inexperienced nurse consult an experienced nurse for validation of the diagnosis. Considering the consequences of inaccurate diagnoses, a consultation is wise before the interventions are set in motion.

Summary

This chapter discussed the evolution of the diagnostic process based on the information processing theory. The multiple steps in the diagnostic process model were presented and examples discussed.

The importance of increasing the accuracy of a nursing diagnosis was stressed and is in fact the focus of this book. Finally, the potential sources of diagnostic error were presented.

In spite of the seeming complexity of the diagnostic process, fear of inaccuracy or diagnostic error must not prevent the nurse from making nursing diagnoses. The degree of accuracy will increase as the nurse's experience and knowledge increase.

Case Studies

Four

Getting Started

In this chapter, beginning-level case studies are presented. The two primary purposes of these cases are to teach you the diagnostic reasoning process and to focus on the diagnostic task.

In the critical thinking activities of these cases you will learn how to differentiate subjective from objective data and how to cluster cues both by functional health patterns and by clustering data from more than one pattern based on general problems. After you have studied several cases in this format, you will have the opportunity to practice the differentiation, organization, and clustering on your own, using cases that are somewhat more complex.

In these beginning cases you will also learn how to generate diagnostic hypotheses, and you will have an opportunity to practice ways of preventing common diagnostic errors. Emphasis is placed on how to determine the most accurate nursing diagnosis.

Through your active participation in working with these cases, we expect that you will:

- Develop sound critical thinking skills
- Apply previously introduced information
- Have an increased awareness of the importance of data collection
- Gain skill in diagnostic reasoning
- Develop the ability to write an accurate diagnostic statement

Mrs. Angela Garcia is a 46-year-old Hispanic woman who works as an x-ray technician at a busy local hospital. She is being seen in the orthopedic clinic for complaints of steadily worsening pain in her right knee. The pain began 4 months ago when she fell and hyperextended the knee. Mrs. Garcia reports that the pain is more intense with weight-bearing activities, including running, standing, and playing tennis. Because of this, she has been limiting her physical activities. She also reports the recent onset of painful muscle spasms in the right leg, both with activity and at rest. The pain and muscle spasms are disrupting her sleep and making it difficult for her to work. At home she has treated the discomfort with acetaminophen and stretching exercises but has experienced no relief.

On physical examination you notice a marked limp with walking, decreased extension in the right knee, and a reluctance to allow her knee to be touched or manipulated. The knee is slightly swollen and warm to the touch. During x-ray examination of the knee, she grimaces in pain when placed in a kneeling position.

Mrs. Garcia's medical diagnosis is patellar tendonitis, and she is started on a regimen of a nonsteroidal antiinflammatory drug (NSAID). As her nurse, you want to use the most accurate nursing diagnosis as a basis for her nursing care. To begin the process of identifying a nursing diagnosis, you first cluster the significant assessment data by functional health patterns as follows:

Health Perception/Health Management Pattern

1. Previous injury to knee four months ago
2. Steadily increasing pain
3. Medical diagnosis: patellar tendonitis
4. NSAID therapy initiated
5. Has used acetaminophen and stretching exercises without relief

Activity/Exercise Pattern

1. Limiting physical activities as a result of pain
2. Muscle spasms at rest and with activity
3. Working is difficult because of pain
4. Limping

5. Decreased extension of right knee
6. Swelling and warmth in right knee
7. Reluctant to allow manipulation of knee

Cognitive/Perceptual Pattern

1. Pain with weight-bearing activities
2. Painful muscle spasms
3. Facial grimacing during x-ray examination

Sleep/Rest Pattern

1. Interrupted sleep because of pain/muscle spasms

Once the data are clustered by functional health patterns, they can be more easily examined to determine general problem areas. General problems may be suggested by one or more significant cues or by overall dysfunction in a particular functional health pattern. General problems for Mrs. Garcia include the following:

1. Pain
2. Trouble sleeping
3. Limitations in her ability to perform usual activities

The client's general problems are helpful as you proceed to the next level of clustering—the grouping of related pieces of data from across multiple functional health patterns. To recluster the data in this manner, the nurse searches all the functional health patterns for cues related to the general problems of pain, trouble sleeping, and limited ability to perform usual activities. Reclustering cues in this way helps clarify the relationship between the individual pieces of data. Data clustered across functional health patterns are more useful in directing thinking about diagnostic hypotheses than are cues considered individually or clustered only by functional health patterns.

You will notice that some cues are included in more than one cluster. This is because cues frequently have logical connections to more than one set of data. For example, in this case there is a link between the client's pain and her interrupted sleep. There is also a logical connection between her pain and her physical limitations. Therefore pain is included in both data clusters.

The clusters of data that can be identified for this client include the following:

Cluster One (General Problem: Pain)

1. Pain in right knee
2. Pain increases with weight-bearing activity
3. Muscle spasms
4. Medical diagnosis: tendonitis

Cluster Two (General Problem: Trouble Sleeping)

1. Pain in right knee
2. Muscle spasms
3. Interrupted sleep

Cluster Three (General Problem: Limited Ability to Perform Usual Activities)

1. Pain in right knee
2. Limiting physical activities
3. Decreased extension and range of motion (ROM)

Based on the clustered data and the general problems that have been identified for this client, specific diagnostic hypotheses that may be considered include the following:

1. *Pain*
2. *Chronic pain*
3. *Sleep pattern disturbance*
4. *Impaired physical mobility*

Critical Thinking Questions

1. Write the definition and defining characteristics of each of the diagnostic hypotheses listed earlier.

PAIN

Definition: _____

_____

_____

Defining characteristics: _____

_____

_____

CHRONIC PAIN

Definition: _____

_____

_____

Defining characteristics: _____

_____

_____

SLEEP PATTERN DISTURBANCE

Definition: _____

_____

_____

Defining characteristics: _____

_____

_____

IMPAIRED PHYSICAL MOBILITY

Definition: _____

_____

_____

Defining characteristics: _____

_____

_____

2. Based on this information, can any of these diagnoses be eliminated? If you answer yes, explain your rationale.

3. Which of the hypotheses represents the most accurate diagnosis for this client? Explain your choice.

4. Write a complete nursing diagnosis statement for the diagnosis you have selected.

The discussion for this case begins on p. 137.

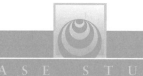

CASE STUDY

Two

Dana Jeffers is a 32-year-old African-American woman being seen in the Women's Health Clinic for an annual physical examination. Her last physical examination and Pap smear were 12 months ago, and she states that she never misses an annual exam. She is a married schoolteacher with no children and describes her current health as "good."

Mrs. Jeffers' history includes a urinary tract infection (UTI) 18 months ago; she has no symptoms at the present time and has not had a recurrence. She reports that she is not using any contraception, since she and her husband hope to conceive their first child in the near future. Her last menstrual period (LMP) was 38 days ago. She has had no previous pregnancies.

This client reports a family history of breast cancer including her mother, her paternal aunt, and her older sister. Although she states that she performs a breast self-examination (BSE) every month, she says she is not confident that she would be able to detect a mass. She requests information on breast cancer prevention and detection strategies, particularly diet and BSE. She also wants to know when she should have her first mammogram.

On physical examination, you find the following: height 5′6″, weight 125 pounds, vital signs within normal limits, breasts soft and nontender with no palpable masses or nipple discharge.

To begin the process of nursing diagnosis, the significant assessment data are first clustered by functional health patterns as follows:

Health Perception/Health Management Pattern

1. Family history of breast cancer
2. Performs BSE monthly
3. Annual pelvic and breast examinations
4. Requesting information on breast cancer detection and prevention
5. Considers current health "good"

Nutritional/Metabolic Pattern

1. Height and weight within normal limits

Elimination Pattern

1. Previous UTI; currently asymptomatic

Activity/Exercise Pattern

1. Vital signs within normal limits

Sexuality/Reproductive Pattern

1. Not using contraception
2. Wants to become pregnant
3. LMP 38 days ago
4. No breast masses, tenderness, or discharge

Not every piece of assessment data provided in the case study is listed as part of the significant data. For example, the patient's age, marital status, and occupation were omitted, since they were not considered relevant diagnostic cues in this situation. Which data are considered significant is a clinical judgment made by the nurse and varies from case to case and with the experience level of the individual clinician. The more experienced nurse may be able to make initial judgments about the significance of cues as the data are collected. Novice nurses are generally unable to make decisions about data this early in the diagnostic process and may not determine which cues are significant until after they cluster the data. Either approach is acceptable; use the method that best suits your experience level and diagnostic style.

From the data that you have organized by functional health patterns, several general problem areas can be identified. These include the following:

1. Family history of breast cancer/need for prevention and detection information
2. Possible pregnancy
3. Previous UTI

Once the general problems have been identified, reclustering the data across functional health patterns helps to further narrow the diagnostic focus. The data can be reclustered as follows:

Cluster One (General Problem: Family History of Breast Cancer/Need for Prevention and Detection Information)

1. Family history of breast cancer
2. Performs BSE monthly; not confident about abilities
3. Receives regular pelvic and breast examinations

4. No breast masses, tenderness, or discharge now
5. Requesting information about BSE, diet, and mammography

Cluster Two (General Problem: Previous UTI)

1. UTI 18 months ago
2. No current symptoms of UTI

Cluster Three (General Problem: Possible Pregnancy)

1. LMP 38 days ago
2. Not using contraception
3. Wants to become pregnant

Based on these clusters, diagnostic hypotheses for this client might include the following:

1. *Health-seeking behaviors: Breast cancer prevention and detection*
2. *Fear* (of developing breast cancer)
3. *Risk for infection (UTI)*

Pregnancy is not listed as a diagnostic hypothesis, even though there are clustered data related to possible pregnancy. This client is 38 days past her LMP, sexually active, and not using contraceptives, so pregnancy is certainly a possibility. However, pregnancy in and of itself is not a nursing diagnosis. An individual client's responses to pregnancy may lead to the identification of nursing diagnoses, but no data either to confirm the pregnancy or to evaluate the client's response to pregnancy are given in this case study. The possibility of pregnancy is a significant collaborative issue. It must be considered by both the nurse and the primary health-care provider in evaluating her breast examination (because of the breast changes associated with pregnancy) and in making a recommendation regarding mammography.

Critical Thinking Questions

1. Write the definition and defining characteristics for each diagnostic hypothesis listed earlier.

HEALTH-SEEKING BEHAVIORS

Definition: _____

_____

_____

Defining characteristics: _____

_____

_____

FEAR

Definition: _____

_____

_____

Defining characteristics: _____

_____

_____

RISK FOR INFECTION

Definition: _____

_____

_____

Defining characteristics: _____

_____

2. Based on this information, can any of these diagnoses be eliminated? If you answer yes, explain your rationale.

3. Which of the hypotheses represents the most accurate diagnosis for this client? Explain your choice.

4. Write a complete nursing diagnosis statement for the diagnosis you have selected.

The discussion for this case begins on p. 138.

Three

Michael Martinez is a 24-year-old Marine who was involved in a motor vehicle accident (MVA) while on leave. His face hit the dashboard, resulting in a fracture of the mandible. Surgery was performed and involved an intermaxillary fixation (wiring of the jaw). As a result of this surgery, he is unable to open his mouth. After surgery he is limited to a liquid diet. This restricted diet will be necessary for 4 to 5 weeks until the fracture heals.

As the nurse responsible for Michael's care, you want to use the most accurate nursing diagnoses as a basis for his care. To begin the process of diagnosis, you review the assessment information and organize the significant assessment data under the appropriate functional health patterns as follows:

Health Perception/Health Management Pattern

1. MVA while on leave
2. Intermaxillary fixation

Nutritional/Metabolic Pattern

1. Intermaxillary fixation
2. Limited to liquid diet for four to five weeks
3. Unable to open mouth

Activity/Exercise Pattern

1. Unable to open mouth

Once the data are clustered according to functional health patterns, the data should be reexamined to determine what general problem areas are suggested by these cues. Three general problems are apparent for this client. This client has problems related to the possibility of aspiration, inadequate nutrition, and breathing.

At this point you are ready to proceed to the next level of clustering. Look at all the cues and ask yourself: What cues are logically associated with the identified problem areas? Clustering cues in this way helps clarify the relationship between the individual pieces of data. Data clustered across functional health patterns are more useful in directing thinking about diagnostic hypotheses than are cues considered individually or clustered only by functional health patterns. Now you are ready to recluster the cues into these general problem areas that you have identified.

Cluster One (General Problem: Possibility of Aspiration)

1. Intermaxillary fixation
2. Unable to open mouth

Cluster Two (General Problem: Inadequate Nutrition)

1. Limited to liquid diet for four to five weeks
2. Unable to open mouth

Cluster Three (General Problem: Possibility of Breathing Problems)

1. Intermaxillary fixation
2. Unable to open mouth

Specific hypotheses that could be considered include the following:

1. *Risk for aspiration*
2. *Altered nutrition: Less than body requirements*
3. *Risk for ineffective airway clearance*

Critical Thinking Questions

1. Write the definition and defining characteristics for each diagnostic hypothesis listed earlier.

RISK FOR ASPIRATION

Definition: _____

_____

_____

Risk factors: _____

_____

_____

ALTERED NUTRITION: LESS THAN BODY REQUIREMENTS

Definition: _____

_____

_____

Defining characteristics: _____

_____

_____

RISK FOR INEFFECTIVE AIRWAY CLEARANCE

Definition: _____

_____

_____

Risk factors: _____

_____

_____

2. Based on this information, can any of these diagnoses be eliminated? If you answer yes, explain your rationale.

3. Why do you think the remaining diagnosis is accurate?

4. Write a complete nursing diagnosis statement for the remaining diagnosis.

The discussion for this case begins on p. 139.

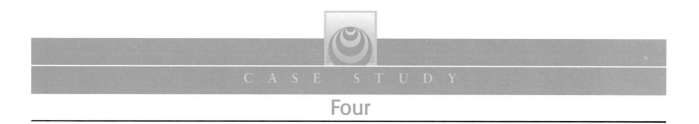

Michael Lovato is a 55-year-old Hispanic man who keeps his appointment with his company's occupational health department for his biannual physical examination. Although he appears to be in generally good health, his current weight is 25% above the ideal weight for his height and frame. His triceps skin-fold measurement is 21 mm (normal 12.5 mm), and his cholesterol level is 245 mg/dl (normal < 200 mg/dl).

His 24-hour dietary recall shows a diet high in fats and low in fruits and vegetables. He states that his lifestyle and job are both sedentary and that he has no regular exercise program. When the nurse brings up the subject of his weight and lack of exercise, he is not opposed to discussing the possibility of losing weight and increasing his exercise.

Critical Thinking Questions

1. List the significant assessment findings.

   Subjective:

   Objective:

2. Organize the significant assessment data by functional health patterns.

3. Using your own words, what general problem areas do you see for this client?

4. Develop data clusters for each of the general problem areas identified in question 3.

5. From the clustered data, develop at least two diagnostic hypotheses using accepted nursing diagnosis labels.

6. Evaluate each of the diagnostic hypotheses by writing and comparing their definitions and applicable defining characteristics.

7. Identify the most accurate nursing diagnosis. Explain your selection.

8. Write a complete nursing diagnosis statement for the diagnosis you have chosen.

The discussion for this case begins on p. 140.

Five

John Chen is an 18-year-old college freshman of Chinese descent. He is being seen in the student health center for follow-up on his complaints of loose, watery stools. When discussing his health history, John states that he has occasionally had some difficulty with diarrhea and has been told in the past that this is due to lactose intolerance. This medical problem has just been confirmed by the student health center physician.

John reports that his diarrhea has worsened over the last 6 months, since the beginning of the school year. He now reports four to six large, loose stools per day with severe abdominal cramping. He reports that his stools are foul smelling and accompanied by a great deal of flatus. He states that he finds this to be a very embarrassing problem, especially while living in a "communal" dormitory situation.

John says that he never drinks milk as a beverage and that when he lived at home he ate a fairly traditional Chinese diet with few milk products. Now that he is eating his meals in the dormitory dining room he feels that he is less able to control the amount of milk products in his diet. Analysis of his 3-day diet recall shows a significant intake of milk products, including cheese, yogurt, and milk-based foods.

On physical examination you find the following: Vital signs and urine specific gravity are within normal limits; height and weight are below average; mucous membranes are pink and moist; skin turgor is normal; capillary refill time is less than 3 seconds; abdomen is soft, with hyperactive bowel sounds.

Critical Thinking Questions

1. List the significant assessment findings.

Subjective:

Objective:

2. Cluster the significant assessment data by functional health patterns.

3. Using your own words, what general problem areas do you see in this case?

4. Develop data clusters for each of the general problems identified in question 3.

5. From the clustered data in question 4, develop at least two diagnostic hypotheses using accepted nursing diagnosis labels.

6. Evaluate each of the diagnostic hypotheses by writing and comparing the definitions and applicable defining characteristics of each diagnosis.

7. Identify the most accurate nursing diagnosis. Explain your selection.

8. Write a complete nursing diagnosis statement for the diagnosis you have chosen.

The discussion for this case begins on p. 142.

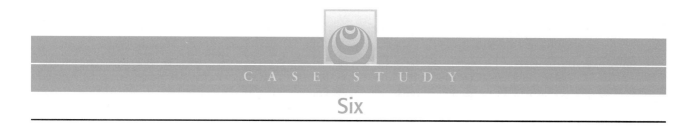

Six

Mrs. Sara Russell is an 84-year-old Caucasian woman admitted to your unit with a diagnosis of breast cancer. She is scheduled for a total mastectomy in the morning. Her surgery has been explained to her, and the consent form has been signed.

Mrs. Russell's admission database indicates a history of a slight hearing loss and poor vision resulting from cataracts. She reports waking each night to void (nocturia). On physical examination you notice cloudy gray cataracts in both eyes. You observe that she has difficulty reading and negotiating her way around the room because of her visual limitations. You also observe that her gait is slow but steady and that she does not use any assistive devices for ambulation.

You have just administered a sedative to help Mrs. Russell sleep. The side rails on the bed are up, and her call light is within reach.

Critical Thinking Questions

1. List the significant assessment findings.

   Subjective:

   Objective:

2. Cluster the significant assessment data by functional health patterns.

3. Using your own words, what general problem areas do you see in this case?

4. Develop data clusters for each of the general problems identified in question 3.

5. From the clustered data in question 4, develop at least two diagnostic hypotheses using accepted nursing diagnosis labels.

6. Evaluate each of the diagnostic hypotheses by writing and comparing their definitions and applicable defining characteristics.

7. Identify the most accurate nursing diagnosis. Explain your selection.

8. Write a complete nursing diagnosis statement for the diagnosis you have chosen.

The discussion for this case begins on p. 144.

James Scofield is a 52-year-old salesman who sustained an accidental gunshot wound of the thigh while on a hunting trip. The postoperative report reveals a traumatic fracture of the right femur with a large area of tissue and muscle damage of the thigh. He had an open reduction and internal fixation (ORIF) of the femur. The wound was cleaned thoroughly by irrigation.

His postoperative medical orders include intravenous (IV) antibiotic administration every 6 hours, administration of pain medication via a patient-controlled analgesia machine (PCA), vital signs every 4 hours for 24 hours, and intravenous fluids to be run at 125 ml per hour for 24 hours, followed by diet as tolerated.

On the patient's admission to your unit, you observe that Mr. Scofield is awake but drowsy; has a large, bulky dressing to his right thigh; has a capillary refill time of 3 seconds in right-side toes; has sensation of touch in right-side toes; has coolness of right-side toes; and can move his toes.

Critical Thinking Questions

1. List the significant assessment findings.

   Subjective:

   Objective:

2. Cluster the significant assessment data by functional health patterns.

3. Using your own words, what general problem areas do you see in this case?

4. Develop data clusters for each of the general problems identified in question 3.

5. From the clustered data in question 4, develop at least two diagnostic hypotheses using accepted nursing diagnosis labels.

6. Evaluate each of the diagnostic hypotheses by writing and comparing their definitions and applicable defining characteristics.

7. Identify the most accurate nursing diagnosis. Explain your selection.

8. Write a complete nursing diagnosis statement for the diagnosis you have chosen.

The discussion for this case begins on p. 146.

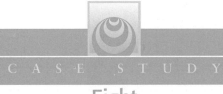

Eight

Joan Stevens is a 20-year-old college student who visits the student health center to have a diaphragm fitted. During the course of the interview she comments that she has a rather embarrassing problem she would like to discuss. On further questioning she tells you that she has a bowel movement accompanied by much straining and effort only every 3 to 4 days. On questioning, you learn that her diet is erratic: meals from a fast-food restaurant are eaten on the run. She walks 3 miles each way to school and back home 5 days a week. She intentionally restricts fluids during the day because of her tight schedule, which precludes regular toilet breaks. She does not use enemas or laxatives because her mother always warned her about developing a laxative dependence.

Your physical examination of Ms. Stevens reveals a well-nourished, trim young woman in apparent good health. Blood pressure is 118/75 mm Hg, pulse rate is 82 beats per minute, respirations are 18 breaths per minute. The examination is unremarkable except for abdominal tenderness on deep palpation. A large mass is palpable in the left lower quadrant of the abdomen.

Critical Thinking Questions

1. List the significant assessment findings.

   Subjective:

   Objective:

2. Organize the significant assessment data by functional health patterns.

3. Using your own words, what general problem areas do you see in this case?

4. Develop data clusters for each of the general problem areas identified in question 3.

5. From the clustered data, develop at least two diagnostic hypotheses using accepted nursing diagnosis labels.

6. Evaluate each of the diagnostic hypotheses by writing and comparing their definitions and applicable defining characteristics.

7. Identify the most accurate nursing diagnosis. Explain your selection.

8. Write a complete nursing diagnosis statement for the diagnosis you selected.

The discussion for this case begins on p. 148.

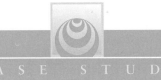

Mr. John Anthony is a 61-year-old man with a history of chronic bronchitis. He has an 80-pack-year smoking history (two packs a day for 40 years). He is being seen in the clinic for complaints of copious thick secretions and the feeling that he is choking on his own sputum. He states that "except for this respiratory problem, my health is good."

Mr. Anthony reports paroxysmal coughing episodes but feels as if he cannot clear his throat, even after coughing. On examination his respiratory rate is 28 breaths per minute and respiration is unlabored; he has bilateral wheezes on auscultation, frequently attempts to clear his throat, and brings up thick yellow mucus with coughing. Mr. Anthony reports that he frequently feels tired in the afternoons and takes a nap after lunch every day. He is independent in all activities of daily living and plays golf three times per week. He eats a well-balanced low-fat diet. He reports a fluid intake of five to six cups of tea or coffee per day and one mixed drink in the evening.

Critical Thinking Questions

1. List the significant assessment findings.

Subjective:

Objective:

2. Cluster the significant assessment data by functional health patterns.

3. Using your own words, what general problem areas do you see in this case?

4. Develop data clusters for each of the general problems identified in question 3.

5. From the clustered data in question 4, develop at least two diagnostic hypotheses using accepted nursing diagnosis labels.

6. Evaluate each of the diagnostic hypotheses by writing and comparing the definitions and applicable defining characteristics of each diagnosis.

7. Identify the most accurate nursing diagnosis. Explain your selection.

8. Write a complete nursing diagnosis statement for the diagnosis you have chosen.

The discussion for this case begins on p. 150.

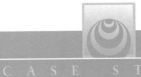

Ten

Georgia Wells, a 71-year-old widow, sustained a left-side hip fracture from a fall in her garden. She has 7 children and 14 grandchildren. She lives in a rural area in a trailer with one of her sons. She has been hospitalized for 3 days and had surgery 2 days ago for a hemiarthroplasty of the left hip. Ms. Wells is very communicative and cooperative. She uses the instructions given to her about positioning related to her hip, such as use of the abductor pillow and avoidance of adduction and hip rotation or flexion greater than 45 degrees.

Ms. Wells reports that her usual weight is 210 pounds, she is 5´8˝ tall. She does not like staying in bed so much and complains of a burning discomfort over her tailbone. Skin on the sacrum is red, and the redness does not resolve after 20 minutes of being off her back. Nurses transfer her from bed to chair three times a day, using both an abductor pillow between her legs and the draw sheet to lift her.

Nurses have documented that she is on a regular diet and has eaten about 70% of all meals. Urinary output has been frequent and in small amounts; total output was 900 ml in the last 24 hours.

Mrs. Wells does not demonstrate any signs of distress over the accident, but she verbalizes a desire to get back to her usual activities. She expresses some concern about the nurse case manager's request that she consider going to a nursing skilled-care facility/rehabilitation center for 3 weeks of physical therapy instead of being discharged directly home. She says she knows she is not able to care for herself yet, but she does not know if she can financially afford to go to a rehabilitation center for such a long time.

Critical Thinking Questions

1. List the significant assessment findings.

   Subjective:

   Objective:

2. Cluster the significant assessment data by functional health patterns.

3. Using your own words, what general problem areas do you see in this case?

4. Develop data clusters for each of the general problem areas identified in question 3.

5. From the clustered data in question 4, develop at least two diagnostic hypotheses using accepted nursing diagnosis labels.

6. Evaluate each of the diagnostic hypotheses by writing and comparing their definitions and applicable defining characteristics.

7. Identify the priority nursing diagnosis. Explain your selection.

8. Write a complete nursing diagnosis statement for the diagnosis selected.

The discussion for this case begins on p. 152.

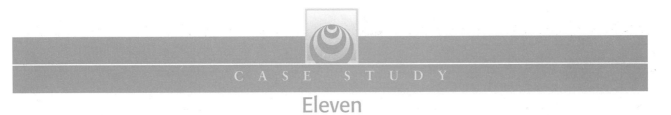

Eleven

Mr. Tafoya, a 26-year-old Hispanic man, states that he is a laborer, employed part-time doing seasonal landscaping work. Two days ago he received second- and third-degree burns to his left arm and hand and second-degree burns to his face, neck, and right arm while lighting trash on fire using gasoline. He rates pain severity as 7 on a scale of 1 to 10. His physician has ordered IV morphine sulfate 2 mg every hour as needed for pain; however, his last pain medication was given 3 hours ago. He complains of nausea from the medication. He also has an order for a regular diet with high-calorie, high-protein supplements, but his observed intake at every meal is less than 30%. He does not drink the supplements. A 24-hour diet analysis reveals that he likes breads and sweets but does not like milk, meat, or cheese. Mr. Tafoya states that he has "always been on the thin side" and is presently 5′10″ tall and weighs 135 pounds. He has lost 3 pounds in the last 24 hours. Laboratory test results reveal a serum albumin level of 2.5 g/dl (normal = 3.5 to 5.0 g/dl).

Critical Thinking Questions

1. List the significant assessment findings.

   Subjective:

   Objective:

2. Cluster the significant assessment data by functional health patterns.

3. Using your own words, what general problem areas do you see in this case?

4. Develop data clusters for each of the general problem areas identified in question 3.

5. From the clustered data in question 4, develop at least two diagnostic hypotheses using accepted nursing diagnosis labels.

6. Evaluate each of the diagnostic hypotheses by writing and comparing their definitions and applicable defining characteristics.

7. Identify the priority nursing diagnosis. Explain your selection.

8. Write a complete nursing diagnosis statement for the diagnosis you selected.

The discussion for this case begins on p. 154.

Five

Building Confidence

The cases in Chapter 5 are more complex than those presented in Chapter 4. The purposes of these cases are as follows:

- To teach you how to write diagnoses for increasingly complex patient situations
- To add the dimension of the situational context
- To provide practice in the identification of priority diagnoses.

At this level the data presented already are clustered by functional health patterns. You will practice identifying highly significant cues (predictive cues) and reclustering the data by general problem areas. Although all functional health patterns are usually assessed, only functional health patterns with significant data are included in each case. Complexity is increased by including in the cases conflicting and disconfirming cues. As you practice these cases, it is hoped that you will refine your ability to efficiently collect data relevant to diagnoses.

The format of the cases presented in this chapter changes slightly from case to case, to focus on different diagnostic challenges. In each case we ask you to identify the general problem areas in the case. In comparing your answers with the answers given, there may be differences. It is expected that as you practice repeatedly you will become more and more precise in pinpointing the general problem areas. An analysis of these differences should also provide excellent discussion material in your classroom setting.

Since this level of cases represents more complex situations, there will always be more than one accurate nursing diagnosis. Often, when there are two or more accurate diagnoses, one emerges as a priority diagnosis. A priority diagnosis is one that should be addressed first, even though other diagnoses are also accurate. In some situations, however, two or more diagnoses have equal priority. These situations are discussed as they are presented. Discussion of the diagnoses clarifies the diagnostic reasoning process and the identification of priority diagnoses.

Twelve

Bill Jones, a 57-year-old man, has had radical neck surgery and a laryngectomy for cancer of the larynx. This is his third postoperative day in the surgical intensive care unit (ICU). He requires frequent oral and tracheostomy suctioning of copious secretions.

Nurses have planned interventions for his *impaired verbal communication* by giving him the call bell, providing a pencil and pad of paper as an alternate means of communication, and asking questions that only require a nod of the head for "yes" or "no."

Assessment Data Clustered by Functional Health Patterns

Health Perception/Health Management Pattern

1. 30-pack-year smoking history
2. Exercised at a gym twice a week before admission

Nutritional/Metabolic Pattern

1. Height 5´10˝; weight 190 pounds
2. Intravenous 5% dextrose in water, 125 ml per hour
3. Tube feedings, 3000 calories per day, by continuous drip through nosogastric tube

4. Questions when he can eat regular food
5. Communicates that he cannot swallow because of his tracheostomy tube

Activity/Exercise Pattern

1. Coughs frequently because of copious secretions

Sleep/Rest Pattern

1. Unable to sleep because of frequent suctioning and routine environmental noise in ICU
2. Reports being very tired

Cognitive/Perceptual Pattern

1. Reports oral pain
2. Morphine sulfate 1 mg per patient-controlled analgesia (PCA) machine for pain

Self-concept/Self-perception Pattern

1. Expresses disgust with his appearance
2. Cries when his wife visits; writes he is sorry he looks so horrible for her

Role/Relationship Pattern

1. Wife very supportive
2. Children visit frequently
3. No friends have been in to see him

Critical Thinking Questions

1. What are the general problem areas that you see for this client?

2. Recluster the data for each of the general problem areas identified in question 1.

3. Do you need to obtain additional data in any of the general problem areas before making a diagnosis?

4. List the diagnostic hypotheses for this case.

5. Look up the definitions and defining characteristics for each diagnostic hypothesis. Based on this information, eliminate inaccurate hypotheses and identify the accurate diagnoses.

6. What are the priority diagnoses for this case?

7. Write the priority diagnoses as complete nursing diagnoses.

The discussion for this case begins on p. 156.

Mrs. Crane is a 60-year-old woman who had multiple coronary artery bypass graft (CABG) surgery 4 days ago. Until the time of her emergency surgery, she was unaware that she had coronary artery disease (CAD). She had some difficulty with respiratory function post-operatively but has been extubated for the last 2 days. She has been moved out of the ICU to the cardiac step-down unit.

You are caring for Mrs. Crane on the night shift. She was awake at 8 PM when you performed her initial assessment and remains awake at midnight. The following database has been developed for Mrs. Crane.

Assessment Data Clustered by Functional Health Patterns

Health Perception/Health Management Pattern

1. Thought she had "stomach problems" until the time of admission; had been self-medicating with antacids
2. Admitted with severe chest pain, shortness of breath, and diaphoresis; angiogram revealed greater than 75% occlusion in multiple coronary arteries
3. CABG surgery performed on day of admission (4 days ago)
4. History of breast cancer 10 years ago
5. Smokes, 20-pack-year history

Nutritional/Metabolic Pattern

1. Weight, 22% above ideal
2. Reported diet was high-calorie, high-fat before surgery
3. Currently eating small amounts of a low-fat diet

Activity/Exercise Pattern

1. Reluctant to move; ambulates to chair and bathroom with much encouragement
2. Complains of being too tired to perform self-care or to ambulate
3. Vital signs within normal limits
4. Breath sounds equal and clear
5. Sedentary lifestyle before surgery; states that "my only exercise is cleaning house"

Sleep/Rest Pattern

1. Awake most of night; dozing at midnight but awakened for vital signs
2. States that she feels exhausted and sleepy
3. Sleeps for short intervals after pain medication is administered
4. States that "I can't sleep with all the noise and activity around here"
5. Dozes off while talking with family
6. States that she is too tired to meet with the dietitian to discuss discharge teaching about nutrition or to attend discharge class for CAD clients
7. States that "I'm afraid to go to sleep"

Cognitive/Perceptual Pattern

1. Requests pain medication every 6 to 8 hours for incisional discomfort
2. States that pain is relieved by pain medication
3. Occasionally slightly confused when asked day or time

Self-concept/Self-perception Pattern

1. States that "I've been a smoker for 20 years, I won't be able to quit now"

Role/Relationship Pattern

1. Husband and three children visit most of the day; they leave at about 9 PM
2. Husband and children ask many questions about client's status and what they can do to help her recover
3. Eldest daughter and husband will help at home after discharge

Critical Thinking Questions

1. What general problem areas can you identify for this client?

2. Develop data clusters for each general problem that you identified in question 1.

3. From your reclustered data, identify at least three diagnostic hypotheses.

4. Review the definitions and defining characteristics for each diagnostic hypothesis. Are there any additional assessment data you would like to collect before ruling each hypothesis in or out?

5. Write all the accurate nursing diagnoses for this client as complete nursing diagnoses.

6. Which is the priority nursing diagnosis? Why?

The discussion for this case begins on p. 159.

Fourteen

Jimmy Lyle is a 32-year-old Native American man who sustained multiple fractures in a motor vehicle accident (MVA). He had surgery 3 days earlier and remains hospitalized.

Assessment Data Clustered by Functional Health Pattern

Health Perception/Health Management Pattern

1. MVA 3 days ago
2. Bilateral tibia and fibula fractures
3. Open reduction, internal fixation (ORIF) of both legs 3 days ago; legs casted
4. Denies tobacco or drug use; states that he drinks a beer occasionally
5. Has a history of juvenile rheumatoid arthritis

Nutritional/Metabolic Pattern

1. Has had no appetite since accident
2. Eats 25% of his meals
3. Feeds himself using adapted utensils
4. Height 5′6″; weight 135 pounds

Elimination Pattern

1. Voids every 3 to 4 hours; urine clear, yellow
2. Had first bowel movement in 3 days today

Activity/Exercise Pattern

1. Significant deformities include enlarged joints of fingers, wrists, elbow, knees, and ankles
2. Used two canes to walk before this accident
3. Has started physical therapy to learn how to walk with crutches
4. Has decreased strength in arms as a result of arthritis
5. Vital signs within normal limits

Sleep/Rest Pattern

1. Feels well rested most of the time

Cognitive/Perceptual Pattern

1. Complains of leg pain; rarely asks for medication
2. States that he has learned how to live with chronic pain resulting from arthritis
3. Holds on to the sides of his legs protectively
4. Speaks English and Navajo

Role/Relationship Pattern

1. Married and has eight children (age range 2 to 12 years)
2. Family members visit and ask questions about how to help him at home
3. Unable to work outside of home because of arthritis
4. Minimal income as self-employed jeweler

Critical Thinking Questions

1. Based on the data presented, what are the general problem areas for this client?

2. Recluster the pertinent data according to the general problem areas identified in question 1.

3. Do you need to obtain additional data in any of the general problem areas before making a diagnosis?

4. List the diagnostic hypotheses for this case.

5. Look up the definitions and defining characteristics for the diagnostic hypotheses before selecting the accurate nursing diagnoses. Based on this information, do you need to eliminate any of the diagnostic hypotheses?

6. What are the priority diagnoses for this client? Write as complete nursing diagnoses.

The discussion for this case begins on p. 162.

Fifteen

Helen Jameson is a 52-year-old woman who has a diagnosis of chronic lymphocytic leukemia. She has been coming to the Cancer Treatment Center for chemotherapy for the past 3 months.

Assessment Data Clustered by Functional Health Patterns

Health Perception/Health Management Pattern

1. Had considered herself to be in good health until leukemia was diagnosed
2. Obtains regular health examinations
3. Has received three courses of chemotherapy, each lasting for 5 days and separated by 6 weeks

Nutritional/Metabolic Pattern

1. "Not eating well since cancer diagnosis"
2. Height 5′7″; weight 140 pounds
3. Ten-pound weight loss before diagnosis
4. Reports episodes of nausea and vomiting after chemotherapy
5. Alopecia resulting from chemotherapy

Elimination Pattern

1. Voids five to six times a day; no change since diagnosis
2. Usually has one bowel movement per day; no change since diagnosis

Activity/Exercise Pattern

1. Used to work full-time and exercise aerobically every other day
2. Has not been back to work since hospitalization because of fatigue

3. Feels very tired; therefore has not been able to exercise
4. Performs self-care

Sleep/Rest Pattern

1. Sleeps 6 to 8 hours per night
2. Takes one to three short naps during the day

Cognitive/Perceptual Pattern

1. Denies any pain
2. Vision and hearing are unchanged
3. Reports being unable to think clearly or concentrate

Self-perception/Self-concept Pattern

1. Viewed herself as an attractive woman before she lost her hair
2. States that she does not want to look at herself now that she has lost her hair
3. Expresses concern that her husband will not love her anymore
4. Cries when she discusses her appearance

Role/Relationship Pattern

1. Husband very affectionate and supportive of wife
2. Husband encourages his wife to put on her makeup as usual and to consider wearing head scarves if she would like to do that

1. What general problem areas can you identify for this client?

2. Develop data clusters for each general problem that you identified in question 1. What additional data do you need in each cluster before you can generate a diagnosis?

3. From your clustered data, identify at least three diagnostic hypotheses.

4. Review the definitions and defining characteristics for each diagnostic hypothesis.

5. List all of the accurate nursing diagnoses as complete statements.

6. Which is the priority diagnosis? Why?

The discussion for this case begins on p. 164.

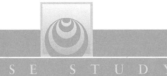

Sixteen

Mrs. Schwartz is a 79-year-old woman who comes to the Genitourinary Clinic with a complaint of dribbling of urine.

Assessment Data Clustered by Functional Health Patterns

Health Perception/Health Management Pattern

1. Considers herself to be in good health
2. Negative Pap test result within the last 6 months

Nutritional/Metabolic Pattern

1. Limits fluid intake in attempt to decrease dribbling
2. Skin dry, prolonged tenting
3. Mucous membranes dry
4. Perineum red and irritated

Elimination Pattern

1. Loses small amount of concentrated urine when lifting grandchildren, coughing, or laughing
2. Wears perineal pad to keep from soiling clothing
3. Slight odor of urine on body and clothing

Activity/Exercise Pattern

1. Restricts activities involving lifting or straining

Sleep/Rest Pattern

1. Gets up two to three times during the night to void
2. Awakens refreshed

Cognitive/Perceptual Pattern

1. Complains of burning in perineal area when urinating

Self-perception/Self-concept Pattern

1. Feels "like a baby" when she leaks urine
2. Is reluctant to leave home for fear that urine smell will offend someone

Role/Relationship Pattern

1. Has two daughters, five grandchildren
2. Has husband of 55 years

Sexuality/Reproductive Pattern

1. Experienced menopause at 50 years of age
2. Has not taken any type of hormone replacement therapy

Critical Thinking Questions

1. Based on the data presented, what are the general problem areas for this client?

2. Recluster the pertinent data according to the general problem areas identified in question 1.

3. List the diagnostic hypotheses for this client.

4. After examining the clustered data and the diagnostic hypotheses, are there any additional questions you would like to ask or assessments you would like to perform?

5. Based on the definitions and defining characteristics, can any of your diagnostic hypotheses be eliminated? If yes, why?

6. Of the remaining hypotheses, which ones are accurate?

7. Write the priority diagnosis as a complete nursing diagnosis.

The discussion for this case begins on p. 167.

Seventeen

Mr. Mark Stevens is a 56-year-old widower with a long history of insulin-dependent diabetes mellitus (IDDM). He was admitted via the emergency department 2 days ago in diabetic ketoacidosis (DKA). His condition is now stable, and he has recently been transferred to the general medical unit. The following nursing database has been developed for Mr. Stevens.

Assessment Data Clustered by Functional Health Patterns

Health Perception/Health Management Pattern

1. IDDM since the age of 15 years
2. Admitted twice with DKA in the last 2 months, last admitted two days ago; IDDM previously well controlled with no DKA admissions or chronic complications associated with IDDM
3. His late wife always helped him check his blood glucose level and administer his insulin
4. States that his biggest problem is that he sometimes forgets to check his blood glucose level and take his insulin
5. States that he does not like being in the hospital and will try to control his diabetes more carefully

Nutritional/Metabolic Pattern

1. Eats more than half of his meals outside the home (restaurants or his children's homes)
2. States that his wife used to do all the cooking
3. Able to verbalize basic principles of American Diabetic Association (ADA) diet
4. Reports that he doesn't always think before he eats
5. Weight within normal range

Elimination Pattern

1. Reports no difficulty with bowel or bladder function

Activity/Exercise Pattern

1. Used to walk two miles every day with wife
2. Used to bowl twice a month with wife
3. Has not walked, bowled, or exercised since wife's death

Cognitive/Perceptual Pattern

1. States that he feels angry and sad about wife's death
2. Reports that he frequently feels "foggy" and has had difficulty making even simple decisions over the last 2 months
3. Alert and oriented
4. Able to verbalize basic principles of diabetes and associated care

Self-perception/Self-concept Pattern

1. Describes himself as a "sad and lonely old man"

Role/Relationship Pattern

1. Married for 30 years
2. Wife died in a motor vehicle accident (MVA) 2 months ago
3. Reports a good relationship with his two children, both of whom live in town and visit him regularly
4. Has five grandchildren
5. Reports that his friends call him every week to go bowling, but he "just doesn't feel like going yet"

Coping/Stress-tolerance Pattern

1. Usually solved problems by discussing them with his wife
2. Tends to eat when he gets sad or worried

Value/Belief Pattern

1. Continues to attend a Methodist church weekly

Critical Thinking Questions

1. What general problem areas can you identify for this client?

2. Develop data clusters for each general problem that you identified in question 1.

3. From your reclustered data, identify at least two diagnostic hypotheses. Are any collaborative problems evident from your data clusters?

4. Review the definitions and defining characteristics for each diagnostic hypothesis. Are there any additional assessment data you would like to collect before ruling each hypothesis in or out?

5. Which is the most accurate nursing diagnosis for this client? Explain your choice.

6. Write a complete nursing diagnosis for the diagnosis you have selected as most accurate.

The discussion for this case begins on p. 169.

Eighteen

Mrs. Harper is an 84-year-old woman with decreasing visual acuity as a result of macular degeneration.

Assessment Data Clustered by Functional Health Patterns

Health Perception/Health Management Pattern

1. Considers health good, except for vision problem

Nutritional/Metabolic Pattern

1. Having increasing difficulty preparing food because of decreased vision
2. Afraid to walk to store to purchase food
3. Many bruises on arms and legs from "bumping into everything"

Elimination Pattern

1. Occasional incontinence resulting from difficulty maneuvering in strange environments and locating toilet

Activity/Exercise Pattern

1. Restricting activity more and more because of fear of falling

Cognitive/Perceptual Pattern

1. Visual acuity, 20/200 with glasses
2. No central vision
3. Very fearful of falling

Self-perception/Self-concept Pattern

1. States that she "feels old and useless"
2. Fears being a burden to family

Role/Relationship Pattern

1. Stays home almost all the time; becomes irritable when family encourages an outing

Critical Thinking Questions

1. Based on the data presented, what are the general problem areas for this client?

2. Recluster the pertinent data according to the general problem areas identified in question 1.

3. List the diagnostic hypotheses for this client.

4. Are there any additional questions you would like to ask or assessments you would like to perform?

5. Based on the definitions and defining characteristics, can you eliminate any of your diagnostic hypotheses? If yes, why?

6. Of the remaining hypotheses, which ones are accurate?

7. Write the priority nursing diagnosis in this case as a complete nursing diagnosis. Explain your selection.

The discussion for this case begins on p. 172.

Today you are making a home visit to Lola Sanders, a 75-year-old woman who was discharged from the hospital yesterday. Her medical diagnosis is heart failure. She is also receiving treatment for mild depression.

Assessment Data Clustered by Functional Health Patterns

Health Perception/Health Maintenance Pattern

1. Rarely goes to doctors
2. Has been under a doctor's care for heart failure for the past 2 months
3. Does not know name or action of two pills she takes daily
4. When she is not symptomatic, she does not take her Lasix on a daily basis

Nutritional/Metabolic Pattern

1. Prepares her own meals three times a day
2. Eats foods from all food groups in amounts recommended by the food pyramid guidelines
3. Does not like to drink fluids because she is "always in the bathroom"

Elimination Pattern

1. States that she feels like she spends the whole day in the bathroom and her bladder always feels full
2. Voids frequently, small amounts with occasional dribbling
3. Palpable bladder

Activity/Exercise Pattern

1. Attended Senior Center three mornings a week for line dancing
2. Experiences dyspnea on exertion, so she stopped dancing
3. Experiences difficulty breathing when in recumbent position

Sleep/Rest Pattern

1. Takes frequent rests during the day
2. Does not sleep well because of difficulty breathing when she lies down
3. Needs two pillows when supine to breathe easily

Self-concept/Self-perception Pattern

1. Is very depressed that she is "in this condition"
2. States that "I never thought I'd have to stop dancing"
3. States that "if this is not going to get any better, I do not want to go on"
4. Family reports that she seems very upset most of the time
5. Takes Elavil 100 mg per day for depression

Role/Relationship Pattern

1. Widow for 8 years
2. Sisters live next door and help with care
3. Son checks on her regularly

Coping/Stress-tolerance Pattern

1. Prays frequently to help her through tough times
2. Admits she does not know what to do now that heart failure has developed

Critical Thinking Questions

1. What are the general problem areas for this client?

2. Recluster the pertinent data according to these general problem areas.

3. List the diagnostic hypotheses for this client.

4. Review the definitions and defining characteristics for each diagnostic hypothesis. Are there any additional assessment data you would like to collect before ruling each hypothesis in or out?

5. Write complete nursing diagnoses for the diagnoses selected.

6. What is the priority diagnosis for this client?

The discussion for this case begins on p. 174.

Twenty

Mrs. Maureen Doyle is a 29-year-old Caucasian woman who is married and has a 3-month-old son and a 3-year-old daughter. She had an abdominal cholecystectomy yesterday. The following database has been developed for Mrs. Doyle.

Assessment Data Clustered by Functional Health Patterns

Health Perception/Health Management Pattern
1. No previous health problems
2. Began complaining of severe epigastric pain radiating to right side 2 days before surgery; cholelithiasis was confirmed by abdominal ultrasound
3. Client has adequate health insurance

Nutritional/Metabolic Pattern
1. Taking sips of water only
2. IV fluids infusing at 125 ml per hour
3. Temperature within normal limits
4. Skin soft with ready recoil; moist mucous membranes

Elimination Pattern
1. Absent bowel sounds
2. No flatus
3. Abdomen moderately distended
4. Complains of nausea
5. Voiding adequate amounts

Activity/Exercise Pattern
1. Reluctant to ambulate because of incisional pain
2. Respiratory rate 26 breaths per minute; respirations shallow
3. Breath sounds clear but diminished bilaterally
4. Refuses to take a deep breath or to use the incentive spirometer because of pain
5. Pulse rate within normal limits

Cognitive/Perceptual Pattern
1. States that "I'm afraid to take a deep breath—it will hurt"
2. Reports nausea, abdominal tenderness, and incisional pain
3. Complains of breast discomfort; has been unable to breast-feed her 3-month-old since surgery
4. Morphine sulfate by patient-controlled analgesia (PCA)

Self-perception/Self-concept Pattern
1. States that "I should be home with my children, not sick in this hospital bed"
2. States that "I'm afraid my baby will forget me"

Role/Relationship Pattern
1. Married; two children (ages 3 months and 3 years)
2. Homemaker; does not work outside the home
3. Belongs to a young-mothers' group at her church
4. States that "I haven't been away from either of my children since they were born"
5. States that "being a good mother is the most important thing I can do"
6. Her husband and her mother are caring for the children while she is hospitalized

Sexuality/Reproductive Pattern
1. Three months postpartum
2. Breastfeeding; has not been able to breastfeed baby since surgery

Coping/Stress-tolerance Pattern
1. Crying intermittently since admission; states that this is because she does not want to be away from her children
2. Is worried about her mother caring for her two children; says "that's my job"
3. Is worried that her children will "think I deserted them"

Critical Thinking Questions

1. What general problem areas can you identify for this client?

2. Recluster the data by the general problem areas that you identified in question 1. Are there any additional assessment data you would like to collect?

3. From your reclustered data, identify at least three diagnostic hypotheses and one collaborative problem.

4. Review the definitions and defining characteristics for each diagnostic hypothesis. Can you confirm or eliminate any diagnoses? If yes, why?

5. Write all the accurate diagnoses for this client as complete nursing diagnoses.

6. Which are the priority diagnoses? Why?

The discussion for this case begins on p. 177.

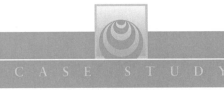

C A S E   S T U D Y

Twenty-One

John Sinclair is a 64-year-old man with a diagnosis of chronic obstructive pulmonary disease (COPD), heart failure, and cor pulmonale. You make a home visit and gather the following information.

Assessment Data Clustered by Functional Health Patterns

Health Perception/Health Management Pattern
1. Considers himself to be in poor health
2. Unable to have oxygen refilled because of lack of money
3. Has COPD, heart failure, and cor pulmonale

Nutritional/Metabolic Pattern
1. Seven-pound weight gain in last 10 days
2. Has 2+ peripheral edema
3. Has an enlarged liver
4. Eats a high-salt diet
5. Advised to follow a diet low in salt with restricted fluids
6. Takes a diuretic each morning

Activity/Exercise Pattern
1. Complains of dyspnea and cough
2. Low-flow oxygen prescribed for nighttime use
3. Full, bounding pulse
4. Hematocrit, 59% (normal for male, 40% to 54%); hemoglobin, 21 g/dl (normal for male, 13.5 to 15.8 g/dl)

Role/Relationship Pattern
1. Unemployed
2. Receiving disability pay for 2 years

Critical Thinking Questions

1. Based on the data presented, what are the general problem areas for this client?

2. Recluster the pertinent data according to the general problem areas identified in question 1.

3. List the diagnostic hypotheses for this client.

4. Are there any additional questions you would like to ask or assessments you would like to perform to refute or corroborate the diagnostic hypothesis?

5. Based on the definitions and defining characteristics, can you eliminate any of your diagnostic hypotheses? If yes, why?

6. Of the remaining diagnoses, which ones are accurate?

7. Write the priority diagnosis for this client as a complete nursing diagnosis.

The discussion for this case begins on p. 180.

Twenty-Two

Arlene Hilton is a 34-year-old woman who was admitted to the hospital with a medical diagnosis of thrombophlebitis of the left femoral artery following an outpatient cardiac catheterization that was performed 4 days ago.

Assessment Data Clustered by Functional Health Patterns

Health Perception/Health Management Pattern

1. Considered herself in good health before diagnosis of mitral stenosis
2. Has a history of rheumatic fever
3. Has had increasing weakness over the past 4 months

Nutritional/Metabolic Pattern

1. Lost 4 pounds in the past week
2. Has dry skin and mucous membranes
3. Complains of thirst

Elimination Pattern

1. Urinating large amounts of dilute urine

Activity/Exercise Pattern

1. Resting blood pressure 94/58 mm Hg
2. Postactivity blood pressure 98/72 mm Hg

Critical Thinking Questions

1. Based on the data presented, what are the general problem areas for this client?

2. Recluster the pertinent data according to the general problem areas identified in question 1.

3. List the diagnostic hypotheses for this client.

4. Based on the definitions and defining characteristics, can you eliminate any of your diagnostic hypotheses? If yes, why?

5. Are there any collaborative problems present in this case?

6. Write the priority diagnoses as complete nursing diagnoses.

The discussion for this case begins on p. 182.

Twenty-Three

Mr. Thomas is a 44-year-old man who is seen in the clinic for complaints of fatigue, anorexia, and insomnia. He is a schoolteacher and spends all of his non-working time caring for his wife, who is terminally ill with ovarian cancer. During his examination he frequently apologizes for yawning. The following database has been developed for Mr. Thomas.

Assessment Data Clustered by Functional Health Patterns

Health Perception/Health Management Pattern
1. Perceives health as "OK"

Nutritional/Metabolic Pattern
1. States that he has not felt hungry since his wife's condition worsened 3 months ago
2. Reports eating coffee and toast for breakfast and no lunch; eats "a little" dinner on the days when his wife is doing fairly well and no dinner on his wife's "bad days"; eats small snacks throughout the day
3. Eight-pound weight loss in the last 3 months; current weight is 9% below ideal
4. Drinks six to eight glasses of water per day
5. Mucous membranes are moist and pink
6. No bruising, rashes, or skin breakdown noted
7. No unusual hair loss reported
8. Has dark circles under his eyes

Activity/Exercise Pattern
1. Used to jog every day; hasn't jogged in 3 months since his wife's condition worsened
2. Lifts weights 30 minutes per day in home gym
3. Rarely goes out anymore, since his wife is too sick to go anywhere
4. Reports feeling tired
5. Has full range of motion and appropriate muscle tone

Sleep/Rest Pattern
1. Sleeps approximately 4 hours per night
2. Has difficulty falling asleep; lies in bed for 1 to 2 hours before falling asleep
3. Reports that his mind "just goes around and around" thinking about his wife's impending death and this keeps him awake
4. Unable to nap during the day; says "I just can't relax enough; every time I lay down I start to cry"

Cognitive/Perceptual Pattern
1. Expresses himself clearly
2. Plans to use home hospice nursing services as wife's condition deteriorates
3. Verbalizes anger over his wife's condition

Self-perception/Self-concept Pattern
1. States that he feels good that he is able to keep his wife at home and do most of her care; feels he is being a good husband

Role/Relationship Pattern
1. States that his wife has been his best friend since they were 16 years old
2. States that he used to tell his wife everything but he is now afraid to talk with her about his feelings, sadness, and fears
3. Wife's family is supportive and helps with her care

Sexuality/Reproductive Pattern
1. No sexual activity; states that his wife is too ill and he isn't really interested anyway; states that "I have more important things to think about"

Coping/Stress-tolerance Pattern
1. Talks to his brother when really angry or sad
2. Verbalizes that he knows his life will never be the same after his wife's death
3. Says "I have no idea how I will cope with this"

Value/Belief Pattern
1. Attends church intermittently; finds comfort in attending
2. Feels that God will help him survive
3. Church members are a source of support for him

Critical Thinking Questions

1. What general problem areas can you identify for this client?

2. Recluster the data by the general problem areas that you identified in question 1.

3. From your reclustered data, identify at least three diagnostic hypotheses for this client.

4. Review the definitions and defining characteristics for each diagnostic hypothesis. Can you confirm or eliminate any hypotheses? If yes, why?

5. List all the accurate nursing diagnoses for this client.

6. Which is the priority diagnosis? Why?

7. Write the priority diagnosis as a complete nursing diagnosis.

The discussion for this case begins on p. 184.

Jane Lucero is a 51-year-old woman who has had full responsibility for the care of her 83-year-old mother, who has had Alzheimer's disease for the past 8 years. On a routine visit to the Geriatric Clinic you have the opportunity to talk to Ms. Lucero about her role as caregiver. During this exchange, you gather the following information about Ms. Lucero.

Assessment Data Clustered by Functional Health Patterns

Health Perception/Health Management Pattern

1. Has not had a Pap test for 6 years
2. Has never had a mammogram
3. Has no chronic illnesses

Nutritional/Metabolic Pattern

1. Eats a high-starch, high-sugar diet
2. Is 22% above ideal body weight

Activity/Exercise Pattern

1. Complains of overwhelming sense of fatigue
2. Has no regular exercise program
3. Has no complaints of dyspnea on exertion
4. Is having increasing difficulty carrying out necessary daily activities

Cognitive/Perceptual Pattern

1. Complains of constant, dull headache
2. Experiences occasional inability to concentrate

Role/Relationship Pattern

1. Quit work 6 years ago to care for mother full-time
2. Has no relief from caregiving responsibilities
3. Has no time or energy to pursue social relationships

Critical Thinking Questions

1. Based on the data presented, what are the general problem areas for this client?

2. Recluster the pertinent data according to the general problem areas identified in question 1.

3. List the diagnostic hypotheses for this client.

4. Are there any additional questions you would like to ask or assessments you would like to perform to refute or corroborate a diagnostic hypothesis?

5. Based on the definitions and defining characteristics, can you eliminate any of your diagnostic hypotheses? If yes, why?

6. Of the remaining hypotheses, which ones are accurate?

7. Write the complete priority nursing diagnosis for this case.

The discussion for this case begins on p. 186.

Six

Gaining Expertise

In Chapter 6 some of the more complex issues in diagnosis are introduced, including the following:

- Identifying personal bias in analyzing data
- Evaluating the accuracy of the nursing diagnosis
- Recognizing the limits of personal knowledge
- Broadening your perspective to include the family as client
- Moving beyond the obvious data to more subtle data

In this chapter, close attention will be paid to you, the diagnostician. Through the questions posed, you will be guided to examine each of these more complex issues.

These cases include more complicated biophysical and psychosocial issues. The format of the cases requires you to consider new data and to substantiate your responses with evidence from reference books.

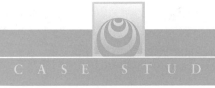

Twenty-Five

Roger Winter is a 33-year-old man with stage III(B) Hodgkin's disease. He has recently been discharged from the hospital following placement of a right atrial catheter to provide long-term central venous access for the chemotherapy he is receiving. The hospital staff has taught him how to care for his catheter, including changing the cap, performing heparin flushes, and changing the dressing. You are seeing this client in the Oncology Clinic to check on his ability to care for the central-line catheter and to administer his second dose of chemotherapy. Mr. Winter's wife, Victoria Jacobsen, is also present during this visit. The following database has been developed for this client.

Assessment Data Clustered by Functional Health Patterns

Health Perception/Health Management Pattern

1. States that he has not felt well for the last 6 months, having symptoms of fatigue, weight loss, and fever that led to his seeking health care
2. Diagnosed with stage III(B) Hodgkin's disease
3. Has mediastinal lymph node involvement and involvement of the spleen
4. Adequate health insurance and medical leave

Nutritional/Metabolic Pattern

1. Height 5′11″; weight before illness of 180 pounds
2. Weight loss of 20 pounds in the 6 months before diagnosis; additional weight loss of 4 pounds since his first chemotherapy treatment
3. Nausea and vomiting for 2 days following last dose of chemotherapy; decreased appetite since then
4. Reports difficulty swallowing

Elimination Pattern

1. No changes in elimination pattern

Activity/Exercise Pattern

1. Reports shortness of breath with activity and at rest
2. Has had a nonproductive cough for several months
3. Hemoglobin 10 g/dl; hematocrit 30%
4. Performs basic activities of daily living but has been unable to work for several weeks because of fatigue, weakness, and shortness of breath
5. Heart rate and respiratory rate within normal limits at rest; become elevated with activity

Sleep/Rest Pattern

1. Reports feeling very tired even though he "sleeps all the time"
2. No difficulty falling asleep at night or napping during the day

Cognitive/Perceptual Pattern

1. Verbalizes a basic understanding of his illness, treatment, and prognosis
2. States that he is very hopeful that treatment will be successful and that he expects to make a full recovery

Self-perception/Self-concept Pattern

1. Says "I am tougher than this disease"
2. Concerned that he is not doing his share of household and family duties; says "I feel like I'm not being a very good husband or father lately; I wish my wife would let me do more things for myself instead of babying me so much"

Role/Relationship Pattern

1. Married for 8 years; has one child
2. Identifies a support system that includes his wife and child, his brother, his mother, and several friends from work
3. He is an architect, currently on medical leave of absence
4. His wife works full time as an accountant

Sexuality/Reproductive Pattern

1. Would like to have more children
2. Has experienced a decrease in libido and sexual activity as a result of fatigue, weakness, shortness of breath, and nausea
3. Reports that his change in sexual activity, concerns about his ability to have more children following chemotherapy, and need to use birth control during treatment are "the worst part of this whole thing"

Coping/Stress-tolerance Pattern

1. Using visualization exercises as an adjunct therapy
2. Finds talking with friends and family helps him cope with his illness

3. Feels that getting back to work will help him cope and is anxious to do this
4. States that he isn't quite used to caring for his central line yet and that he would like his wife to also learn how to care for the line
5. Says that his wife is more worried about his illness than he is and that she is always fussing or worrying about everything since his diagnosis

Value/Belief Pattern

1. Does not attend church or belong to any organized religion
2. Believes he must actively help in making himself well
3. Would like to try nontraditional healing methods but his wife says these methods are silly and a waste of time and energy

Critical Thinking Questions

PART ONE

1. What factors increase the complexity of this client's situation?

2. Consider the context in which this client interaction takes place (the setting, purpose of the interaction, and so forth). Has the nurse collected the appropriate assessment data? Are there any additional data you feel should be collected even before the identification of problem areas and diagnostic hypotheses?

See discussion on p. 189 before proceeding.

PART TWO

1. Based on both the original data and the new data, what general problem areas can you identify? Recluster all the data according to these general problems.

2. Generate as many diagnostic hypotheses as possible for Mr. Winter and his family.

3. Examine each hypothesis. Which diagnoses are accurate in this case?

4. Do you have any personal beliefs or biases that may have influenced your diagnostic reasoning in this case?

5. How would you select priorities for this client? Identify your highest priority diagnoses.

6. Write complete nursing diagnoses for all the priority diagnoses you have selected.

The discussion for Part Two begins on p. 190.

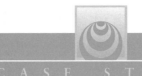

Part One

John Martin is a 59-year-old man who was brought into the Salvation Army shelter at 11 PM. You are a student nurse who is at the shelter as part of your community health rotation. You proceed to gather basic health and social information from this man as part of the intake for all shelter clients. During the course of the assessment you gather the following information.

Assessment Data Clustered by Functional Health Patterns

Health Perception/Health Management Pattern

1. Non–insulin-dependent diabetes mellitus (NIDDM) for past 8 years
2. States that health is "OK"
3. Reluctant to discuss lifestyle and health habits
4. Not currently taking any medication for diabetes
5. Wearing jeans and a sweatshirt
6. Poorly groomed with strong body odor
7. Random blood sugar level of 648 mg/dl
8. Had been living under viaduct until brought into shelter

Nutritional/Metabolic Pattern

1. Height 5′11″; weight 145 pounds
2. Skin parched, lips dry
3. Eats one meal a day at local homeless shelter
4. Blood pressure 96/64 mm Hg; temperature 97.1° F; pulse rate 112 beats per minute; respirations 12 per minute
5. Draining 5- by 7-cm lesion on malleolus of right foot
6. Refuses offer of a snack, stating that he has no appetite

Elimination Pattern

1. Urinated two times during 30-minute assessment
2. No ketones on dipstick urinalysis

Activity/Exercise Pattern

1. Lethargic and hypoactive
2. Able to ambulate without assistance

Cognitive/Perceptual Pattern

1. Grimaces when abdomen is palpated
2. Able to follow requests
3. Unable to read Consent to Treat form without glasses, which he lost

Self-perception/Self-concept Pattern

1. Very passive in interactions with shelter personnel
2. Will not attempt physical response to examination requests (such as, "touch your nose"), says "I can't"
3. Avoids eye contact with interviewer
4. Sits with shoulders slumped, hands hanging at sides

Role/Relationship Pattern

1. When asked about family and work, states that "they've all given up on me"

Coping/Stress-tolerance Pattern

1. Says "I'm a loner"

Value/Belief Pattern

1. States that "God gave up on me a long time ago"
2. Repeatedly apologizes that time and resources are going to a "bum like me"

Additional information related to the context and diagnostician have particular relevance to this case and must be considered. These factors include the following:

Contextual Factors

1. Salvation Army shelter not equipped to treat acutely ill clients
2. Two other paid nonprofessional staff are present at the facility but are very busy with other clients
3. Outside temperature is 22° F
4. Clients usually stay at facility for only 1 to 3 nights

Diagnostician Factors

1. Student nurse is a senior at nearby university
2. Able to reach supervising faculty at all times via phone
3. Finds this client offensive
4. Feeling very rushed with three other clients waiting to be processed through the admission procedure before they can get a meal and a bed

Critical Thinking Questions

PART ONE

Perhaps many of you can identify with the student nurse in this situation. She is caring for a very complex client with multiple physical and social problems in a less than ideal setting. Resisting her initial reaction to panic, she quickly sets about trying to organize a large amount of data. She asks herself the following question:

1. What are the general problem areas for this client?

Because she has identified so many problem areas and recognized the possibility of an emergency, she knows she has to focus more on the client's medical situation. She decides to prioritize the general problem areas even before she hypothesizes about nursing diagnoses. She believes that unless she eliminates some of the less urgent problems, her care will be too scattered to accomplish anything meaningful.

2. Of the problem areas identified earlier, what areas will you address at this time?

3. Recluster the appropriate data into the problem areas identified in question 1.

Now that the large database has been pared down to a manageable amount and the most important problem areas have been identified, the nurse can generate appropriate nursing diagnoses.

4. What are the nursing diagnoses appropriate for this client?

5. Examine each hypothesis. Which diagnoses are accurate in this case?

6. Do you recognize any biases on the part of the student nurse that could interfere with her diagnostic reasoning?

The discussion for Part One begins on p. 194.

Twenty-Six

Part Two

Following his treatment at the Salvation Army Shelter, Mr. Martin was hospitalized for 10 days. On his admission to the hospital, a nursing conference was held to establish diagnoses and plan interventions for this very ill man. Ms. Demarest, an experienced nurse who has worked on the unit for several years, took an interest in Mr. Martin and cared for him consistently during his hospitalization. Many of the positive changes in his life, particularly those relating to his lifestyle, were made as a result of Ms. Demarest's interest and perseverance. During this time, Mr. Martin's diabetes was brought under control. The following data are current at discharge.

Assessment Data Clustered by Functional Health Patterns

Health Perception/Health Management Pattern

1. Has a small wardrobe provided from hospital clothing bank, including a heavy winter coat
2. States that "I don't ever want to be that sick again"
3. Had extensive teaching regarding management of his diabetes
4. Concerned about his ability to maintain his prescribed treatment plan
5. Glyburide 10 mg/day prescribed
6. Random blood sugar 130 mg/dl (normal 70–120 mg/dl, fasting)
7. Clean and well groomed
8. Has been accepted into local halfway house for room, board, and job retraining

Nutritional/Metabolic Pattern

1. Discharge weight 154 pounds (9 pound gain)
2. Placed on 2500-calorie diabetic diet
3. Lesion on right foot healing well with no signs of inflammation

Activity/Exercise Pattern

1. Able to perform all self-care activities without assistance
2. Ambulating without problems

Cognitive-Perceptual Pattern

1. No abdominal pain
2. Reads easily with glasses from Lion's Club Eyeglass Bank

Self-perception/Self-concept Pattern

1. Makes many denigrating remarks about himself and homeless state
2. States that "I need to get out of here to make room for someone who deserves all this attention"

Role/Relationship Pattern

1. Had no visitors during his hospitalization
2. Made no phone calls

Coping/Stress-tolerance Pattern

1. Unwilling to discuss his life or the events leading to his homelessness
2. Coping styles appear to be denial and avoidance

Value/Belief Pattern

1. Refused to see hospital chaplain
2. States that "God gave up on me a long time ago"

To formulate a discharge summary and provide direction for the nurse who will be following up Mr. Martin in the community, another care conference was held. The purpose of this conference was to identify the nursing diagnoses in need of interventions.

Critical Thinking Questions

PART TWO

1. What are the general problem areas for this client at discharge?

2. Recluster the appropriate data into the identified problem areas.

Ms. Demarest took charge at the discharge conference. She wrote the following diagnostic hypotheses on the chalkboard and stated that "these are the diagnoses which we'll enter on Mr. Martin's transfer sheet:"
   a. *Ineffective management of therapeutic regimen related to complex care requirements as manifested by expressed concern over ability to manage prescribed treatment plan*
   b. *Altered nutrition: Less than body requirements related to thin appearance as manifested by undernourished appearance*
   c. *Self-esteem disturbance related to homeless state as manifested by self-denigrating comments*
   d. *Altered family process related to nonsupportive family as manifested by lack of family visits*
   e. *Ineffective individual coping related to unknown etiology as manifested by use of denial and avoidance*
   f. *Spiritual distress related to homeless state as manifested by refusal to see hospital chaplain and comment about God giving up on him*

3. As a participant in the discharge conference, you requested that each diagnosis be considered individually. You cared for Mr. Martin on numerous occasions and believed that several of these diagnoses were not accurate. Discuss the accuracy of each nursing diagnosis made by Ms. Demarest.

4. Summarize the errors made by Ms. Demarest in her critical thinking about Mr. Martin.

5. List the nursing diagnoses that you would include on the discharge summary.

6. Write the priority nursing diagnosis for this client.

The discussion for Part Two begins on p. 197.

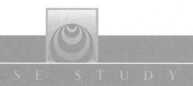

Twenty-Seven

Part One

Eileen Mitchell, 22 years old, had a skiing accident at 16 years of age, which resulted in paraplegia from a T1 vertebral fracture. Your home visit today is for the purpose of changing the dressing on an ischial pressure ulcer.

Assessment Data Clustered by Functional Health Pattern

Health Perception/Health Management Pattern

1. Skiing accident 6 years ago resulting in paraplegia
2. 22-year-old woman
3. Lives alone in an apartment complex adapted for handicapped adults
4. Bedroom dark, curtains drawn, clutter all over the room and many piles of soiled clothing and linen

Nutritional/Metabolic Pattern

1. Stage-IV ischial pressure ulcer
2. An empty can of Coke and a box of cookies at her bedside

Elimination Pattern

1. Ureterostomy
2. Bag full of urine; full urinal at bedside
3. Urine clear yellow
4. Incontinent of a very large, loose, unformed stool
5. Usually manages bowel continence with diet modification and bowel evacuation schedule

Activity/Exercise Pattern

1. Paraplegic; uses wheelchair
2. Has taken care of herself "as long as I can remember"
3. Lying supine in bed with pillows surrounding her

Role/Relationship Pattern

1. Works as a bookkeeper
2. Has no friends
3. Mother lives in town but only comes by "once in a while"
4. Has sign on door saying "Do not bother me!"

Self-concept/Self-perception Pattern

1. Disheveled, unkempt

Value/Belief Pattern

1. Goes to Baptist church "most Sundays"

Critical Thinking Questions

PART ONE

1. Identify factors that increase the complexity of this case.

2. Based on the data presented, what are the general problem areas for Ms. Mitchell?

3. Recluster the pertinent data according to the general problem areas identified in question 2.

4. What questions would you ask to obtain the additional data needed to make a diagnosis?

Read discussion on p. 199 before continuing with Part Two questions.

Critical Thinking Questions

PART TWO

1. Based on your analysis of all the data, what are the diagnostic hypotheses for this client?

2. Analyze your diagnostic hypotheses, and write complete nursing diagnoses for the priority diagnoses.

3. How does the context of the client-nurse interaction affect your analysis?

The discussion for Part Two begins on p. 201.

Discussion

1 and 2. *Pain* is defined as "a state in which an individual experiences and reports the presence of severe discomfort or an uncomfortable sensation."[3] The defining characteristics include verbal and/or nonverbal communications of pain, guarding, a self-focus or narrowed focus, use of distraction behaviors, facial expressions of pain, and physiologic changes such as increased heart rate or diaphoresis. Mrs. Garcia exhibits many of these symptoms; this remains a viable diagnostic hypothesis.

By definition, *chronic pain* lasts for at least 6 months. Since this client's pain has been present for only 4 months, *chronic pain* can be eliminated as a diagnosis.

Impaired physical mobility is "a state in which the individual experiences a limitation of ability for independent physical movement."[3] The defining characteristics include the inability to move within the physical environment (including bed mobility, transfer, and ambulation), limited ROM, and decreased muscle strength or control. While Mrs. Garcia has pain with movement and has elected to limit some activities, she still is capable of independent movement within her environment. She does not have decreased muscle control or limited ROM. Therefore *impaired physical mobility* is not an accurate diagnosis and can be eliminated from consideration.

Sleep pattern disturbance occurs when the "disruption of sleep time causes discomfort or interferes with desired lifestyle."[3] Defining characteristics include difficulty falling asleep, awakening earlier than desired, interrupted sleep, and complaints of not feeling well rested. This client does complain of interrupted sleep, but there is no evidence that tiredness is causing problems for her. Her problems are caused by pain, not by interrupted sleep. *Sleep pattern disturbance* would be a low-accuracy diagnosis in this case.

3. The nursing diagnosis *pain* is the most accurate diagnosis for this client at this time. Her presenting signs and symptoms include verbal complaints of pain, difficulty in weight-bearing because of pain, guarding of the knee, and facial grimacing when placed in a kneeling position. These cues support the diagnosis of *pain* for Mrs. Garcia.

4. A complete nursing diagnosis for this client is as follows: *Pain related to swelling of right knee, weight-bearing activities, and unsuccessful self-management as manifested by report of pain, difficulty in weight-bearing, and failure to gain relief from acetaminophen and stretching.* The diagnostic statement can be further clarified by adding a "secondary to" statement, which links the nursing diagnosis to the pathology or medical diagnosis. The complete diagnosis would then be as follows: *Pain related to inflammation, weight-bearing activities, and unsuccessful self-management secondary to traumatic injury and tendonitis as manifested by report of pain, difficulty in weight-bearing, warmth and swelling of right knee, and failure to gain relief from acetaminophen and stretching.*

Case Study Two

1 and 2.   The definition of the nursing diagnosis *fear* is "a feeling of dread related to an identifiable source which the person validates."[3] The defining characteristic is the ability to name the object of fear. The client may also exhibit feelings of dread or apprehension, avoidance behaviors, and concentration on danger, as well as physiologic indicators of distress such as increased heart rate, shortness of breath, and sweating. None of these behaviors are present in Ms. Jeffers; therefore *fear* is not an accurate diagnosis. Although it may be reasonable to expect that a woman with a family history of breast cancer would be fearful of developing this disease, there are no data available to confirm this suspicion. Ms. Jeffers does not make any comments about being afraid of developing cancer; she only discusses her desire to prevent and detect it.

Risk for infection (UTI) can be eliminated, since it is not a highly accurate diagnosis in this case. The definition of *risk for infection* is "the state in which an individual is at increased risk for being invaded by pathogenic organisms."[3] The defining characteristics are the risk factors that make a person highly susceptible to infection; these include interrupted skin barrier, stasis of body fluids (such as urine), anemia, immunosuppression, and chronic disease. Although Ms. Jeffers has had one previous UTI, there are no data to suggest that she is at increased risk for development of another infection. No risk factor such as urinary tract abnormality or predisposing condition is identified in the case study. Risk diagnoses should not be used indiscriminately as catch-all diagnoses. They should be used only when the individual client's risk is unique or greater than the risk expected for most people. Although the nurse will always be alert for signs and symptoms of a UTI, to assign the diagnosis *risk for infection* would be inappropriate for this client.

As defined by NANDA, *health-seeking behavior* is "the state in which an individual in stable health is actively seeking ways to alter personal health habits and/or the environment in order to move toward a higher level of health."[3] The major defining characteristic is the client's expressed desire to seek a higher level of wellness. The expression of concern about current health is also a defining characteristic. This remains a viable diagnostic hypothesis for Ms. Jeffers.

3.   The most accurate diagnosis for this client is *health-seeking behaviors: Breast cancer prevention and detection.* Ms. Jeffers' concern over her family history of breast cancer, along with her request for more information about BSE, mammography, and cancer prevention diets, is clearly consistent with the definition and defining characteristics of this diagnosis. Based on her family history, her identification of this as an area of concern, and her lack of other urgent health problems, this health-related issue is a priority diagnosis for this client.

4.   The priority nursing diagnosis for this client is correctly written as a one-part statement: *Health seeking behaviors: breast cancer prevention and detection.* An etiologic statement (or "related to" statement) would be redundant and is not necessary with the diagnosis *health-seeking behaviors.*

Case Study Three

1, 2, and 3. *Risk for aspiration* is defined as "the state in which an individual is at risk for entry of gastrointestinal secretions, oropharyngeal secretions, or solids or fluids into tracheobronchial passages."[3] There are many defining characteristics for this nursing diagnosis, such as reduced level of consciousness, depressed cough and gag reflexes, presence of tracheostomy or endotracheal tube, and wired jaw. The most relevant defining characteristic is wired jaw. Because of the presence of this highly relevant cue, it is highly accurate to assign this nursing diagnosis to Mr. Martinez.

Another diagnosis worth considering for this client is *risk for ineffective airway clearance*. This diagnosis is defined as "a state in which an individual is unable to clear secretions or obstructions from the respiratory tract to maintain airway patency."[3] Relevant defining characteristics include abnormal breath sounds, rhonchi, changes in rate or depth of respiration, cyanosis, and dyspnea.

The nursing diagnosis of *risk for ineffective airway clearance* is very close to the diagnosis *risk for aspiration*. In this case, although the definitions for both diagnoses are appropriate and fit the clinical situation, the defining characteristics suggest selecting *risk for aspiration*. Careful analysis of the defining characteristics indicate that *risk for aspiration* is usually associated with a mechanical restriction problem, whereas *risk for ineffective airway clearance* is more commonly used when respiratory secretions are the problem. Here is a case in which both diagnoses are accurate and would direct different, but equally appropriate, nursing interventions. However, knowledge of specific characteristics, as well as clinical experience and judgment, shifts the balance to selection of *risk for aspiration* as the guiding nursing diagnosis.

The remaining nursing diagnosis under consideration for this client is *altered nutrition: Less than body requirements*. This diagnosis is defined as "the state in which an individual experiences an intake of nutrients insufficient to meet metabolic needs."[3] Relevant defining characteristics include loss of weight with adequate food intake, body weight 20% or more under the ideal, reported inadequate food intake less than the Recommended Daily Allowance (RDA), and weakness of muscles required for swallowing or mastication.

At this time it is possible to rule out the nursing diagnosis of *altered nutrition: Less than body requirements*. There is no evidence to support this diagnosis in the present clinical situation. However, because it is possible that the patient could have a problem maintaining his present weight and avoiding weight loss, the diagnosis of *risk for altered nutrition: Less than body requirements* could be considered an appropriate diagnosis. This diagnosis would direct nursing interventions to the prevention of the problem of weight loss. Careful planning by the nurse and the dietitian could keep this patient in excellent nutritional state. As time passes and the client adjusts to his nutritional and eating limitations, additional assessment information would indicate whether this nursing diagnosis could be eliminated or made an actual diagnosis.

The nursing diagnosis *risk for aspiration* is an important diagnosis that will direct the nurse to be vigilant while Michael has wires in place. It is also a highly important diagnosis because of the consequences of aspiration.

4. A complete nursing diagnosis for this case would be as follows: *Risk for aspiration related to inability to open mouth secondary to intermaxillary fixation.* (Remember, defining characteristics are not included in a risk diagnosis. Only the diagnostic category and the etiologic statement are necessary.)

Case Study Four

1. The significant assessment findings include the following:

Subjective

1. Diet high in fats and low in fruits and vegetables
2. Sedentary job and lifestyle
3. No regular exercise program
4. Not opposed to discussing possibility of losing weight and increasing exercise

Objective

1. Weight 25% above ideal for height and frame
2. Triceps skin-fold measurement, 21 mm
3. Serum cholesterol level, 245 mg/dl

2. The assessment data are organized under the following functional health patterns:

Health perception/health management pattern

1. Not opposed to discussing possibility of losing weight and increasing exercise

Nutritional/metabolic pattern

1. Diet high in fats and low in fruits and vegetables
2. Weight 25% above ideal for height and frame
3. Triceps skin-fold measurement, 21 mm
4. Serum cholesterol level, 245 mg/dl

Activity/exercise pattern

1. Sedentary job and lifestyle
2. No regular exercise program

3. The general problem areas are as follows:

a. Weight above ideal body weight
b. Poor nutritional habits
c. Sedentary lifestyle

4. These data can be reclustered as follows:

Cluster One (general problem: Weight above ideal body weight and poor nutritional habits)

1. Diet high in fats and low in fruits and vegetables
2. Weight 25% above ideal for height and frame
3. Triceps skin-fold measurement, 21 mm
4. Serum cholesterol level, 245 mg/dl
5. Not opposed to discussing possibility of losing weight

Cluster Two (general problem: Sedentary lifestyle)

1. Sedentary job and lifestyle
2. No regular exercise program
3. Not opposed to discussing possibility of increasing exercise

5. Diagnostic hypotheses for this client might include the following:

a. *Altered nutrition: more than body requirements*
b. *Altered health maintenance*
c. *Activity intolerance*
d. *Health-seeking behavior*

6 and 7. The most accurate nursing diagnosis is *altered nutrition: more than body requirements*. This diagnosis is congruent with the definition that it is a "state in which an individual is experiencing an intake of nutrients which exceeds metabolic needs."[3] Relevant defining characteristics include the following: weight 20% over the ideal for height and frame, triceps skin-fold value greater than 15 mm in men, sedentary activity level, and reported or observed dysfunctional eating pattern. Two of the major defining characteristics ("critical characteristics" as labeled by NANDA in Taxonomy I) are present and ensure the accuracy of the diagnosis.

Altered health maintenance might also be considered as a diagnosis. However, the NANDA definition of this diagnosis is "inability to identify, manage, and/or seek out help to maintain health."[3] There are many defining characteristics for this diagnosis. Defining characteristics that might be applicable include the following: Demonstrated lack of knowledge regarding basic health practices, demonstrated lack of adaptive behaviors to internal or external environmental changes, reported or observed inability to take responsibility for meeting basic health practices in any or all functional pattern areas, and history of health-seeking behavior. Based on this definition and these defining characteristics, the diagnosis of *altered health maintenance* is not a highly accurate diagnosis for Mr. Lovato because there is no match between the cues in this case and the defining characteristics for the diagnosis.

Different sources can give alternative definitions and defining characteristics for the same nursing diagnosis. Many authors use the diagnosis of *altered health maintenance* when the presence of risk factors for a specific health problem is noted. In this case the nurse recognizes the presence of risk factors for coronary artery disease. However, *altered nutrition: More than body requirements* is a more accurate diagnosis when using NANDA definition and defining characteristics. If an alternative definition and set of defining characteristics were used, *altered health maintenance* might be the priority nursing diagnosis because of the importance of initiating teaching to reduce the risk factors associated with coronary artery disease, a more significant health problem than obesity alone.

The cues of sedentary job and lifestyle may lead you to consider *activity intolerance* as a diagnosis. *Activity intolerance* is defined as "a state in which an individual has insufficient physiologic or psychologic energy to endure or complete required or desired daily activities."[3] The defining characteristics include verbal report of fatigue or weakness, abnormal heart rate or blood pressure response to activity, exertional discomfort or dyspnea, and electrocardiographic changes reflecting dysrhythmias or ischemia. On close scrutiny it is apparent that there is no match between either the definition or defining characteristics and the data presented. This is a case where the label alone looks like it might match the cues of sedentary job and lifestyle. However, further examination of the definition and defining characteristics indicates that this is not an accurate diagnosis because there are no data to support it.

Health-seeking behavior is defined as "a state in which an individual in stable health is actively seeking ways to alter personal health habits, and/or the environment in order to move toward a higher level of health."[3] The major defining characteristics include the expressed or observed desire to seek a higher level of wellness. The minor defining characteristics are expressed or observed desire for increased control of health practices, expression of concern about the effect of current environmental conditions on health status, stated or observed unfamiliarity with wellness community resources, and demonstrated or observed lack of knowledge in health promotion behaviors. This diagnosis is not accurate because Mr. Lovato is not actively seeking assistance for his weight problem. Although not opposed to the idea of losing weight and increasing his exercise, his lack of initiative on these topics does not support the diagnosis of *health-seeking behavior*. The nurse should be alert to the development of cues supporting the possibility, and if supported by future data, might consider this diagnosis at a later time.

8. The complete nursing diagnosis based on this case is as follows: *Altered nutrition: More than body requirements related to high-fat, low-vegetable and -fruit diet and sedentary lifestyle as manifested by weight 25% above the ideal triceps skin-fold 21 mm, and cholesterol level of 245 mg/dl.*

Case Study Five

1. The significant assessment findings include the following:

Subjective

1. History of diarrhea, worsening over last 6 months
2. History of lactose intolerance
3. Four to six large, loose stools per day
4. Stools are foul smelling, accompanied by flatus and abdominal cramping
5. Reports embarrassment as a result of flatus and odor
6. Does not drink milk as a beverage but diet recall shows significant intake of milk products
7. Eats meals in dormitory cafeteria
8. Ate a traditional Chinese diet with few milk products when he lived at home

Objective

1. Vital signs and specific gravity within normal limits
2. Height and weight below average
3. Mucous membranes pink and moist
4. Normal skin turgor
5. Capillary refill time, less than 3 seconds
6. Abdomen soft
7. Hyperactive bowel sounds

2. The assessment data are clustered under the following functional health patterns:

Health perception/health management pattern

1. History of diarrhea
2. History of lactose intolerance
3. Moved to college 6 months ago

Nutritional/metabolic pattern

1. Does not drink milk as a beverage but diet recall shows significant amounts of milk products in food
2. Eats meals in dormitory cafeteria
3. Height and weight below normal
4. Mucous membranes pink and moist
5. Normal skin turgor
6. Ate a traditional Chinese diet when he lived at home

Elimination pattern

1. Four to six large, loose stools per day
2. Stools are foul smelling and accompanied by flatus and abdominal cramping
3. Abdomen soft

4. Hyperactive bowel sounds
5. Urine specific gravity within normal limits

Activity/exercise pattern

1. Capillary refill time, less than 3 seconds
2. Vital signs within normal limits

Self-perception/self-concept pattern

1. Embarrassed by flatus and odor that accompany stools

3. The general problem areas for John Chen are as follows:

1. Diarrhea
2. Increased consumption of milk products
3. Possible inadequate nutrition
4. Embarrassment

4. These data can be reclustered as follows:

Cluster One (general problem: Diarrhea)

1. History of lactose intolerance
2. Diarrhea worsening over last 6 months
3. Four to six large, loose stools per day
4. Stools accompanied by flatus and abdominal cramping
5. Significant intake of milk products in foods
6. Hyperactive bowel sounds

Cluster Two (general problem: Intake of milk products)

1. History of lactose intolerance
2. Diet recall shows significant intake of milk products in foods
3. Eats meals in dormitory cafeteria
4. Worsening diarrhea since starting school 6 months ago
5. Ate a diet low in milk products before starting college

Cluster Three (general problem: Possible inadequate nutrition)

1. Height and weight below average
2. History of diarrhea, worsening over last 6 months
3. Abdominal cramping
4. Eats most meals in dormitory cafeteria

Cluster Four (general problem: Embarrassment)

1. Reports embarrassment because of flatus and stool odor

5. Diagnostic hypotheses for this client might include the following:

1. *Diarrhea*
2. *Altered nutrition: Less than body requirements*
3. *Situational low self-esteem*

6 and 7. The definition of the nursing diagnosis *diarrhea* is "a state in which an individual experiences a change in normal bowel habits characterized by the frequent passage of loose, fluid, unformed stools."[3] The defining characteristics include increased frequency of stools, loose liquid stools, abdominal pain, cramping, and urgency. This client exhibits almost all of these findings; therefore *diarrhea* is a highly accurate nursing diagnosis for this client. The cluster of data related to his increased consumption of milk products suggests an etiology for this diagnosis.

The diagnosis *altered nutrition: Less than body requirements* is suggested primarily by the cue of height and weight below average. Supporting data that may suggest a cause are the client's diarrhea and abdominal cramping and the fact that he eats his meals in the dormitory cafeteria. However, the definition of this diagnosis is "the state in which an individual experiences an intake of nutrients insufficient to meet metabolic needs."[3] It is not clear from the data given that this is the case. A number of questions must be answered to more fully consider this diagnosis: Has the client actually lost weight, or has his weight been stable? How much "below average" are his height and weight? Might the standard height and weight charts be inappropriate for a person of Chinese ancestry? If so, might his height and weight actually be appropriate for him? Until these questions are answered, the diagnosis *altered nutrition: Less than body requirements* cannot be confirmed and is therefore not an accurate diagnosis.

The final diagnostic hypothesis, *situational low self-esteem*, is based on the client's report of embarrassment caused by the symptoms associated with diarrhea. The definition of *situational low self-esteem* is "negative self evaluation/feelings about self which develop in response to a loss or change in an individual who previously had a positive self-evaluation."[3] The major defining characteristic is expressing negative feelings about oneself in response to a specific life event or verbalizing an episodic negative appraisal of the self. The expression of shame is a minor defining characteristic. This client has only one cue (embarrassment) that is consistent with the diagnosis *situational low self-esteem*. No information about his basic self-concept or a self-appraisal is provided; therefore this is an inaccurate diagnosis.

One diagnosis that is often associated with diarrhea is *fluid volume deficit*. *Fluid volume deficit* is defined as "vascular, cellular, or intracellular dehydration."[3] The defining characteristics include decreased urine volume, concentrated urine, sudden weight loss, hypotension, increased pulse rate and body temperature, decreased skin turgor, and dry mucous membranes. Although this diagnosis is commonly found in association with the nursing diagnosis *diarrhea*, it was not considered as a diagnostic hypothesis in this case. Not only are the defining characteristics for *fluid volume deficit* not present in this client, but also a number of cues clearly conflict with the diagnosis. These conflicting cues include vital signs within normal limits, normal skin turgor, specific gravity within normal limits, and moist mucus membranes. Early recognition of conflicting cues can eliminate a diagnosis from consideration even before the hypothesis generation stage. However, a less experienced nurse may not recognize conflicting cues so early in the diagnostic process and may have listed *fluid volume deficit* as a hypothesis. The hypothesis would then be ruled out when the client's data are compared to the definition and defining characteristics for fluid volume deficit.

8. The most accurate diagnosis for John Chen is correctly written as follows: *Diarrhea related to inability to adhere to prescribed therapeutic diet in dormitory environment as manifested by four to six large, loose stools per day accompanied by abdominal cramping.*

Case Study Six

1. The significant assessment findings include the following:

Subjective

1. Poor vision
2. Slight hearing loss
3. Nighttime voiding (nocturia)
4. Recent admission to hospital

Objective

1. Slow gait
2. Visible cataracts in both eyes
3. Difficulty reading and getting around the room
4. Recent administration of a sedative
5. Breast cancer with impending mastectomy

2. The assessment data are clustered by functional health patterns as follows:

Health perception/health management pattern

1. Breast cancer with impending mastectomy
2. Change in health status (because of illness)
3. Move to hospital environment

Elimination pattern: Nocturia

Activity/exercise pattern

1. Slow gait
2. Difficulty getting around in hospital environment

Cognitive/perceptual pattern

1. Cataracts in both eyes
2. Difficulty in reading
3. Slight hearing loss
4. Recent sedation

3. The general problem areas for Mrs. Russell are as follows:

a. Possible worry about the effects of surgery
b. Safety while in the hospital
c. Poor vision
d. Nocturia

4. These data can be reclustered as follows:

Cluster One (general problem: Possible worry about the effects of surgery)

1. Breast cancer
2. Impending mastectomy
3. Change in health status

Cluster Two (general problem: Safety)

1. Sensory/motor impairments (vision, hearing, gait)
2. Unfamiliar environment
3. Sedation
4. Nocturia

Cluster Three (general problem: Poor vision)

1. History of poor vision
2. Visible cataracts in both eyes
3. Difficulty in reading and getting around the room

Cluster Four (general problem: Nocturia)

1. Nighttime voiding
2. Age, 84 years

5. Diagnostic hypotheses for this client might include the following:

a. *Body image disturbance*
b. *Risk for injury: Falls*
c. *Sensory/perceptual alteration: Visual and auditory*
d. *Altered urinary elimination*

6 and 7. *Risk for injury: Falls* is the most accurate diagnosis for Mrs. Russell because it reflects a serious, immediate threat to her safety. The definition for this diagnosis is "the state in which an individual is at risk of injury as a result of environmental conditions interacting with the individual's adaptive and defensive resources."[3] This definition is consistent with the facts presented in this case.

The presence of risk factors is the defining characteristic for the diagnosis *risk for injury*. The basic risk factors for Mrs. Russell are her decreased visual acuity, nocturia, and slow gait. These risk factors are increased by her admission to the unfamiliar environment of the hospital and further increased by the potential effects of sedation. Nurses have a professional and legal obligation to identify these risks, make this diagnosis, and intervene appropriately.

A second diagnosis, *altered urinary elimination,* can be considered based on the client's report of nighttime voiding. Nocturia is one of the defining characteristics for this diagnosis. The definition of *altered urinary elimination* is "the state in which the individual experiences a disturbance in urine elimination."[3] Nocturia may be a normal age-related change in elimination pattern or may indicate a disturbance for this client. It is not clear from the data given whether the nocturia is a significant problem. No clues to the etiology are given in this case study. Additional data are needed before this diagnosis can be confirmed or eliminated.

The diagnosis *sensory/perceptual alteration: visual and auditory* might also be considered for this client. *Sensory/perceptual alteration* is "a state in which the individual experiences a change in the amount or patterning of oncoming stimuli accompanied by a diminished, exaggerated, distorted or impaired response to such stimuli."[3] Although not inconsistent with the definition, the use of this diagnosis is not useful in guiding nursing care for this client. It may be useful as an etiology. The diagnosis *risk for injury: Falls* accurately describes this client's possible response to her sensory/perceptual deficit.

Several other diagnoses commonly associated with the preoperative mastectomy client may also come to mind. These diagnoses include *anxiety, body image disturbance,* and *anticipatory grieving;* however, no data exist to support any of these diagnoses. Each could be identified as a possible nursing diagnosis for this client. The professional nurse continues to assess for data that support these (and other) additional diagnoses but does not make diagnoses based on generalizations about clients when these diagnoses are not supported by specific assessment findings.

8. This at-risk diagnosis is correctly written as a two-part statement as follows: *Risk for injury: Falls related to unfamiliar environment, visual and auditory deficits, sedation, and history of nocturia.*

Case Study Seven

1. The significant assessment findings include the following:

Subjective

1. Sensation of touch to right-side toes
2. Hunting accident
3. Reports coolness in right foot

Objective

1. Gunshot wound with fracture of right femur and large area of tissue and muscle damage
2. ORIF right femur
3. Large, bulky dressing to right thigh
4. Awake but drowsy
5. Capillary refill time, 3 seconds in right-side toes
6. Moves right-side toes well
7. IV fluids 125 ml per hour for 24 hours
8. Diet as tolerated
9. IV antibiotics every 6 hours
10. PCA for pain
11. Immediate postoperative period
12. Wound cleaned by irrigation (during surgery)

2. The assessment data are clustered under the following functional health patterns:

Health perception/health management pattern

1. Gunshot wound with fracture of right femur; ORIF, femur
2. Accident occurred while hunting
3. Immediate postoperative period
4. Large, bulky dressing to right femur
5. Wound cleaned by irrigation (during surgery)

Nutritional/metabolic pattern

1. IV fluids 125 ml per hour for 24 hours
2. Diet as tolerated
3. IV antibiotics every 6 hours

Activity/exercise pattern

1. Capillary refill time, 3 seconds in right-side toes
2. Motor function intact in right-side toes
3. Toes cool (right foot)

Cognitive/perceptual pattern

1. Sensation intact in right-side toes
2. Using PCA for pain

3. The general problem areas are as follows:
a. Neurovascular function of right leg
b. Possible infection

4. Recluster data to support the general problem areas as follows:

Cluster One (general problem: Neurovascular function of right leg)

1. Gunshot wound with fracture of right femur
2. ORIF, right femur
3. Capillary refill time, 3 seconds in right-side toes
4. Sensation intact in right-side toes
5. Motor function intact in right-side toes
6. Toes cool (right foot)
7. Immediate postoperative period

Cluster Two (general problem: Possible infection)

1. Gunshot wound to right upper leg with fracture of right femur and large area of tissue and muscle damage
2. Accident occurred while hunting
3. ORIF right femur
4. IV antibiotics every 6 hours
5. Wound cleaned by irrigation (during surgery)

5. Based on the clustered data and the general problems that have been identified for this client, the diagnostic hypotheses that may be considered include the following:

a. *Risk for peripheral neurovascular dysfunction*
b. *Risk for infection*

6 and 7. *Risk for peripheral neurovascular dysfunction* is defined by NANDA as "a state in which an individual is at risk of experiencing a disruption in circulation, sensation, or motion of an extremity."[3] Remember that for *risk* diagnoses you must identify the risk factors rather than the defining characteristics. Mr. Scofield presents relevant risk factors for this diagnosis, such as tissue trauma and fractures. As a result of these factors, Mr. Scofield may have localized edema, which would impair his circulation, sensation, or motion of the affected foot. There is some evidence that he has adequate neurovascular function of the foot at this time, such as capillary refill time of 3 seconds, movement, and sensation in the affected toes. The highly relevant cue of coolness of the toes is suggestive of impaired neurovascular function. Therefore, because there is a highly relevant cue and there are risk factors, this diagnosis is accurate as a risk diagnosis at this time. You would treat the client by elevating the foot, encouraging gentle foot movement, and continuing to monitor for signs of impaired neurovascular function.

Risk for infection is defined as "the state in which an individual is at increased risk for being invaded by pathogenic organisms."[3] The most relevant risk factors in this case include broken skin, traumatized tissue, tissue destruction, and increased environmental exposure. This diagnosis is also accurate because of the presence of highly relevant cues.

Mr. Scofield is at risk for both of the preceding nursing diagnoses; however, the nursing diagnosis of *risk for peripheral neurovascular dysfunction* is of paramount importance at this time because it represents the most immediate and serious postoperative threat.

8. A complete nursing diagnosis for Mr. Scofield is *risk for peripheral neurovascular dysfunction related to the effects of extensive tissue trauma*. A risk diagnosis requires only a two-part statement: The label and the risk factors.

Case Study Eight

1. The significant assessment findings include the following:

Subjective

1. Wants to have diaphragm fitted
2. Bowel movement every 3 to 4 days; straining at stool
3. Meals erratic, from fast-food restaurants
4. Restricts fluid intake during day
5. Walks 3 miles a day to school and back

Objective

1. Blood pressure 118/74 mm Hg; pulse rate 82 beats/min; respirations 18 breaths/min
2. Appears well nourished and trim
3. Lower left quadrant (LLQ) tenderness on deep palpation
4. Large palpable mass in LLQ

2. The presented assessment data are organized under the following functional health patterns:

Health perception/health management pattern

1. Requests diaphragm fitting
2. Appears to be in good health

Nutritional/metabolic pattern

1. Well nourished, trim
2. Meals erratic, from fast-food restaurants
3. Restricts fluid intake during day

Elimination pattern

1. Bowel movement every 3 to 4 days; straining at stool
2. Large amount of hard stool palpable in LLQ

Activity/exercise pattern

1. Walks 3 miles per day to school and back
2. Blood pressure 118/74 mm Hg; pulse rate 82 beats/min; respirations 18 breaths/min

Cognitive/perceptual pattern

1. Abdominal tenderness on deep palpation

Value/belief pattern

1. Does not use laxatives or enemas because of mother's advice

3. The general problem areas are as follows:

a. Desire to have diaphragm fitted
b. Constipation
c. Poor food- and fluid-intake habits

4. These data can be clustered as follows:

Cluster One (general problem: Constipation)

1. Bowel movement every 3 to 4 days; straining at stool
2. Restricts fluid intake during day
3. Does not use laxatives or enemas because of mother's advice
4. Abdominal tenderness on deep palpation
5. Palpable mass in LLQ
6. Meals erratic, from fast-food restaurants
7. Walks 3 miles per day to school and home

Cluster Two (general problem: Desire to have diaphragm fitted)

1. Wants to have diaphragm fitted
2. Vital signs within normal limits
3. Apparent good health

Cluster Three (general problem: Poor food- and fluid-intake habits)

1. Meals erratic, from fast-food restaurants
2. Appears to be well nourished and trim

5. Diagnostic hypotheses for this client might include the following:

a. *Constipation*
b. *Altered health maintenance*
c. *Health-seeking behavior*
d. *Fluid volume deficit*

6 and 7. The diagnostic hypotheses proposed for this client should be studied individually to identify the most accurate diagnosis. In this case the most accurate diagnosis is *constipation*. The NANDA definition of *constipation* is "a state in which an individual experiences a change in normal bowel habits characterized by a decrease in frequency and/or passage of hard dry stools."[3] The defining characteristics for *constipation* include decreased activity level; frequency less than usual pattern; hard, formed stools and palpable mass; reported feeling of pressure in rectum; reported feeling of rectal fullness; straining at stool; abdominal pain; appetite impairment; back pain and headache; interference with daily living; and use of laxatives. In Ms. Stevens' case sufficient defining characteristics are present in the assessment data to support this diagnosis. The fact that she walks 3 miles regularly is a conflicting cue for this diagnosis. The usual finding related to activity for this diagnosis is a decreased activity level. However, the strength of the other cues makes this unusual finding irrelevant. Although constipation is not the reason for her entering the health-care system, you would recognize that this is a potentially serious problem and is amenable to nursing interventions.

Health-seeking behavior: Effective contraception is another diagnostic hypothesis worth considering. The NANDA definition for the diagnosis of *health-seeking behavior (specify)* is "a state in which an individual in stable health is actively seeking ways to alter personal health habits and/or the environment in order to move toward a higher level of health."[3] The major defining characteristic is an expressed or observed desire to seek a higher level of wellness. The minor defining characteristics for *health-seeking behavior* include expressed or observed desire for increased control of health practices; expression of concern about current environmental conditions on health status; stated or observed unfamiliarity with wellness community resources; demonstrated or observed lack of knowledge in health promotion behaviors. The major defining characteristic for *health-seeking behavior* is present. However, this diagnosis would not be considered the priority diagnosis because it will be easily resolved at the present clinic visit. Although it is a correct diagnosis, it has a low degree of accuracy (+2; see Table 3-6) because it has a lower priority than other diagnoses.

Health-seeking behavior: Improved nutrition might also be a diagnostic hypothesis. Certainly, the nurse would want to suggest better nutritional practices. However, when considering the definition and defining characteristics as listed in the preceding paragraph, it becomes clear that the major characteristic of actively seeking ways to improve personal health habits

is not present in this case. Ms. Stevens did not initiate the discussion of diet and fluids; this information came out as a result of the nurse's analyzing the symptom of constipation.

To address the data related to food and fluid intake, you might consider the diagnosis of *altered health maintenance*. The NANDA definition of this diagnosis is "inability to identify, manage, and/or seek out help to maintain health."[3] There is no need to look at defining characteristics, since analysis of the definition precludes the use of this diagnosis. The nurse will include appropriate nursing interventions related to diet teaching as part of the plan for *constipation*.

Finally, *fluid volume deficit* may appear to be a logical diagnosis based on the symptom of restricted fluid intake. The NANDA definition for this diagnosis is "the state in which an individual experiences vascular, cellular, or intracellular dehydration."[3] The defining characteristics include change in urine output, change in urine concentration, sudden weight loss or gain, decreased venous filling, hemoconcentration, change in serum sodium level, hypotension, thirst, increased pulse rate, and decreased skin turgor. This is not an accurate diagnosis because neither the definition nor the defining characteristics match the clinical data presented in this case. Ms. Stevens' state of good health and normal vital signs are conflicting cues to this diagnosis.

8. The most accurate diagnosis for the case is correctly written as *constipation related to diet and low fluid intake as manifested by bowel movement every 3 to 4 days, straining at stool, LLQ tenderness* on deep palpation, and palpable mass in LLQ.

Case Study Nine

1. The significant assessment findings include the following:

Subjective

1. Chronic bronchitis
2. 80-pack-year smoking history
3. Sensation of choking on secretions
4. Report of paroxysmal coughing episodes
5. Daily fluid intake of five to six cups of tea and coffee
6. Afternoon tiredness relieved by napping
7. Independent in activities of daily living
8. Plays golf three times per week
9. Health "good" except for respiratory problem

Objective

1. Respiratory rate of 28 breaths/min, unlabored
2. Bilateral wheezes
3. Thick, yellow mucus with coughing
4. Frequent attempts to clear throat

2. The significant assessment data are clustered under the following functional health patterns:

Health perception/health management pattern

1. Chronic bronchitis
2. 80-pack-year smoking history
3. Health "good" except for respiratory problem

Nutritional/metabolic pattern

1. Daily fluid intake of five to six cups of tea or coffee

Activity/exercise pattern

1. Thick, yellow secretions
2. Paroxysmal coughing episodes
3. Bilateral wheezes
4. Increased respiratory rate (28 breaths/min)
5. Independent activities of daily living
6. Golf three times per week

Sleep/rest pattern

1. Afternoon tiredness
2. Nap every afternoon

Cognitive/perceptual pattern

1. Sensation of choking

3. The general problem areas are as follows:

a. Respiratory dysfunction
b. Fatigue
c. Inadequate fluid intake

4. These data can be further clustered as follows:

Cluster One (general problems: Respiratory dysfunction)

1. Chronic bronchitis
2. Smoking (80-pack-year history)
3. Thick, yellow secretions
4. Paroxysmal coughing episodes
5. Sensation of choking on secretions
6. Elevated respiratory rate (28 breaths/min)
7. Low fluid intake (five to six cups of tea or coffee daily)
8. Bilateral wheezes

Cluster Two (general problem: Fatigue)

1. Afternoon tiredness
2. Daily afternoon nap

Cluster Three (general problem: Inadequate fluid intake)

1. Drinks primarily coffee or tea (five to six cups per day)

5. Diagnostic hypotheses for this client might include the following:

a. *Ineffective airway clearance*
b. *Fatigue*
c. *Sleep pattern disturbance*
d. *Altered health maintenance*
e. *Fluid volume deficit*

6 and 7. The most accurate diagnosis in this case is *ineffective airway clearance*. The NANDA definition of *ineffective airway clearance* is as follows: "The state in which an individual is unable to clear secretions or obstructions from the respiratory tract to maintain airway patency."[3] The defining characteristics for this diagnosis include abnormal breath sounds, ineffective cough, abnormal respiratory rate or effort, and cyanosis. At least one of these findings must be present to confirm the diagnosis; it is not necessary that they all be present. Mr. Anthony's chief complaints are all related to airway compromise—he has thick secretions, a sensation of choking on secretions, and coughing that is not effective in clearing the secretions. He also has an elevated respiratory rate. The assessment data clearly support the nursing diagnosis of *ineffective airway clearance*.

Fatigue is an inaccurate diagnosis in this case because the assessment findings are not consistent with the definition and defining characteristics for this diagnosis. The definition of *fatigue* includes the fact that the exhaustion is sustained (unrelieved by rest) and limits physical and mental capacity.[3,11] The inability to maintain usual activities and client report of an overwhelming lack of energy are defining characteristics of *fatigue*. Mr. Anthony does report tiredness, but he is able to effectively manage this with an afternoon nap. He reports no limitations in his activities and continues to play golf regularly.

The diagnosis *sleep pattern disturbance* is similarly incorrect. The definition states that a person has this diagnosis when "a disruption of sleep time causes discomfort or interferes with desired lifestyle."[3] The defining characteristics include difficulty falling or remaining asleep and behavioral changes associated with lack of sleep. These behaviors include such things as irritability, inability to keep one's eyes open, and yawning. Mr. Anthony reports no such difficulties; therefore *sleep pattern disturbance* is an inaccurate diagnosis.

The nursing diagnosis *altered health maintenance* is defined as the "inability to identify, manage, and/or seek out help to maintain health."[3] Defining characteristics include inadequate knowledge of health practices, lack of adaptive behaviors, and not taking personal responsibility for meeting basic health needs. Additional defining characteristics are a lack of resources or social support needed to maintain health.

Several findings in Mr. Anthony's history may support this diagnosis. He has a long-standing smoking history and inadequate fluid intake. He may lack the necessary knowledge to make the connection between his health habits and his current respiratory problems. For example, he may not understand the importance of increased fluid intake in thinning his secretions. He may not realize that coffee and tea are poor fluid choices because they act as diuretics, causing mild dehydration and increasing the thickness of secretions. While *altered health maintenance* is a possible diagnosis for this client, further assessment of his knowledge base is needed before the diagnosis can be confirmed. If the diagnosis is confirmed with further assessment, it is an important, but not the priority, diagnosis for Mr. Anthony. Treatment should be instituted after the client's more immediate needs related to airway clearance are addressed.

Fluid volume deficit is also an inaccurate diagnosis for this client, even though his fluid intake is suboptimal. The definition of this diagnosis is "the state in which an individual experiences vascular, cellular, or intracellular dehydration."[3] The defining characteristics include decreased urine output, hemoconcentration, change in serum sodium level, dry skin, and dry mucous membranes. None of these findings is noted in the assessment data provided. A further assessment of fluid status is warranted with this client, but data are insufficient to support this diagnosis at the present time. Although a diagnosis related to fluid intake cannot be made, Mr. Anthony's low fluid intake is an important cue and suggests an etiology for his airway clearance problem.

8. The most accurate diagnosis for Mr. Anthony is correctly written as follows: *Ineffective airway clearance related to copious thick secretions, smoking, and inadequate fluid intake as evidenced by sensation of choking on sputum, inability to clear secretions with coughing, elevated respiratory rate, and wheezing.*

Case Study Ten

1. The significant assessment findings include the following:

Subjective

1. Reported weight 210 pounds; height 5´8´´
2. Does not like staying in bed so much
3. Complains of burning discomfort over her tail-bone
4. Desires to return to usual activities
5. Concerned about going to rehabilitation center
6. Lives in a trailer with adult son

Objective

1. Widow, 71 years old
2. Hemiarthroplasty of left hip 2 days earlier
3. Communicative and cooperative
4. Uses correct "hip precautions"
5. Sacral redness that does not resolve within 20 minutes
6. Out of bed to chair three times a day with abductor pillow in place
7. Eats 70% of regular diet
8. Urine output 900 ml in frequent, small amounts

2. The data are clustered into the following functional health patterns:

Health perception/health management pattern

1. Widow, 71 years old
2. Lives in trailer with adult son
3. Hemiarthroplasty of left hip 2 days earlier
4. Uses correct "hip precautions"

Nutritional/metabolic pattern

1. Weight 210 pounds; height 5´8´´
2. Regular diet, 70% eaten
3. Sacral redness that does not resolve within 20 minutes

Elimination pattern

1. Urine output 900 ml in frequent, small amounts

Activity/exercise pattern

1. Does not like staying in bed so much
2. Desires to return to usual activities
3. Out of bed three times a day with abductor pillow in place

Cognitive/perceptual pattern

1. Complains of burning discomfort over her tail-bone
2. Communicative and cooperative
3. Concerned about going to a rehabilitation center

3. The general problem areas are as follows:

a. Skin condition
b. Discharge plans
c. Immobility

4. These data can be reclustered as follows:

Cluster One (general problem: Skin condition)

1. Sacral redness that does not resolve within 20 minutes
2. Complains of burning discomfort over tailbone
3. Does not like staying in bed so much
4. Transfer out of bed three times a day with abductor pillow in place and by lifting on the draw sheet
5. Desires to return to usual activities
6. Weight 210 pounds; height 5´8´´
7. Hemiarthroplasty of left hip 2 days earlier

Cluster Two (general problem: Discharge plans)

1. Concerned about going to a rehabilitation center
2. Desires to return to usual activities

Cluster Three (general problem: Immobility)

1. Hemiarthroplasty of left hip 2 days earlier
2. Nurses lift her out of bed three times a day to chair
3. Does not like staying in bed so much

5. Diagnostic hypotheses for this client might include the following:

a. *Impaired skin integrity*
b. *Impaired physical mobility*
c. *Fear*
d. *Decisional conflict*

6 and 7. The priority nursing diagnosis is *impaired skin integrity* because there is already evidence that a skin problem is present and several risk factors are present that will increase the degree of skin impairment if not dealt with. The definition of this diagnosis is "a state in which the individual's skin is adversely altered."[3] The defining characteristic that is present for this client is a disruption of the skin surface, that is, sacral redness that does not resolve within 20 minutes. Related or etiologic factors are that the client is obese, spends a lot of time either in bed or in a chair with pressure on her sacrum.

Impaired physical mobility is also a diagnosis to consider in this situation. The diagnosis is consistent with the definition that it is "a state in which the individual experiences a limitation of ability for independent physical movement."[3] Likewise, a defining characteristic is that the client is unable to move purposefully within the physical environment. Depending on the surgical procedure used to repair her hip fracture, the physician will order specific progression of the client's activity. Regardless of the client's mobility, however, the nurse is primarily concerned about the client's skin. Moreover, *impaired physical mobility* is an etiologic factor for *impaired skin integrity* in this situation.

Fear or *decisional conflict* are two additional nursing diagnoses that are considered. At this point in your thinking, both of these would be possible diagnoses, since data are insufficient to accurately make an actual diagnosis. The nurse should clarify which of the two diagnoses is present by asking about the client's feelings about the discharge to a rehabilitation center. This questioning should elicit whether the "concern" the client has expressed is actually a fear or whether the client is in conflict because she has to choose between rehabilitation or going home without adequate preparation.

This questioning can be done by validating the nursing diagnosis with the client. For example, the nurse may ask, "It seems to me that you may be afraid about going to a rehabilitation center. Is that correct?" or, "Are you having difficulty choosing to go to a rehabilitation center?" Answers to these questions should provide data to confirm or discard one of the diagnoses.

8. The complete priority nursing diagnosis based on this case is as follows: *Impaired skin integrity related to obesity, impaired physical mobility, and pressure on sacrum as manifested by sacral redness which does not resolve within 20 minutes.*

Case Study Eleven

1. Significant assessment findings include the following:

Subjective

1. Pain severity of 7 on a scale of 1 to 10
2. Nausea after pain medication
3. Prefers breads and sweets; dislikes meat, milk, and cheese
4. Has "always been on the thin side"

Objective

1. Second- and third-degree burns to left arm and hand
2. Second-degree burns to face, neck, and right arm
3. Hispanic, 26 years old; height 5′10″; weight 135 pounds
4. Three-pound weight loss in last 24 hours
5. Regular diet with high-calorie, high-protein supplements
6. Eats less than 30% of meals, does not drink supplements
7. Serum albumin level 2.5 g/dl
8. Morphine 2 mg IV every hour as needed
9. Last medicated for pain 3 hours ago

2. The assessment data are organized under the following functional health patterns:

Health perception/health management pattern

1. History of being thin
2. Second- and third-degree burns

Nutritional/metabolic pattern

1. Height 5′10″; weight 135 pounds
2. History of being thin
3. Three-pound weight loss in past 24 hours
4. Nausea after morphine
5. Order for regular diet with supplements
6. 30% of meals eaten; no supplements drunk
7. Serum albumin level 2.5 g/dl
8. Prefers breads and sweets; dislikes meat, milk, and cheese

Cognitive/perceptual pattern

1. Pain severity of 7 on a scale of 1 to 10
2. IV morphine 2 mg every hour as needed
3. Last medicated for pain 3 hours ago

3. The general problem areas are as follows:

1. Inadequate nutritional intake
2. Pain

4. The data are clustered as follows:

Cluster One (general problem: Inadequate nutritional intake)

1. History of being thin
2. Second- and third-degree burns
3. Three-pound weight loss in past 24 hours
4. Nausea after morphine
5. Order for regular diet with supplements
6. 30% of meals eaten; no supplements drunk
7. Prefers breads and sweets; dislikes milk, meat, and cheese
8. Serum albumin level 2.5 g/dl

Cluster Two (general problem: Pain)

1. Second- and third-degree burns
2. Pain severity of 7 on a scale of 1 to 10
3. Morphine 2 mg IV every hour as needed
4. Last medicated for pain 3 hours ago
5. Nausea after morphine

5. Diagnostic hypotheses for this client might include the following:

a. *Altered nutrition: Less than body requirements*
b. *Pain*

6 and 7. *Altered nutrition: Less than body requirements* is the nursing diagnosis of primary concern to the nurse at this stage in the client's recovery. The increased metabolic needs of a burned client necessitate an increased intake of protein and calories to heal the burn and to reduce the risk of infection. This diagnosis is congruent with the definition: The state in which an individual experiences an intake of nutrients insufficient to meet metabolic needs.[3] The defining characteristics in this case are loss of weight, body weight more than 20% under the ideal, and food intake less than the recommended daily allowance.

The etiologies in this diagnosis are not absolutely clear in this case. The nurse would need to validate the etiologies with the client. Etiologies suggested by the data include the pain and nausea. Discussing with the client the relationship of pain and nausea to appetite may also help identify why the client is not eating well, since both pain and nausea can certainly affect one's appetite.

This diagnostic hypothesis can be tested by considering other pieces of data—specifically, the client's admission height and weight, history of always being thin, and serum albumin level. The nurse needs to determine the client's usual nutritional intake. Mr. Tafoya is hypoalbuminemic, which indicates that his intake of protein is very low unless he has an ongoing disease process such as chronic liver disease or collagen vascular disease. Validation of his usual level of protein intake would be helpful in analyzing this situation.

Caloric needs are increased greatly in the burn client because of the hypermetabolic and highly catabolic state resulting from the burn. The nurse must encourage the client to eat high-protein, high-carbohydrate foods to meet his increased caloric needs. The database indicates that this client prefers high-carbohydrate but low-protein foods that have been offered to him. The client may have culturally related food preferences or may lack knowledge about nutritional values of foods, or other factors may be influencing his dietary intake. Exploring his usual food intake will provide the nurse with useful information in individualizing his care.

Pain is also considered as a diagnosis. In the burn client pain is one of the key problems addressed by both the medical and nursing personnel. Since pain treatment is pharmacologic at this early stage of the burn, it is considered a collaborative problem. This collaborative problem would be written as *potential complication: pain*. The nurse would be concerned that Mr. Tafoya rates his pain at 7, which is a relatively high level of pain. This rating, along with the information that he was last medicated 3 hours ago and he feels nauseated after he takes the pain medication, would lead the nurse to wonder several things. Is the client aware of how often he may receive the medication? Does the client have fears about the medication, such as fear of becoming addicted? Is the client avoiding use of the medication because it makes him nauseated? Further assessment is needed to collect enough data to accurately treat his pain.

Nausea should be monitored and treated as a collaborative problem also. Nausea is a fairly common adverse effect of narcotics. Nausea may also be a factor in Mr. Tafoya's low level of food intake. Since treatment of the nausea involves interdependent interventions, it should be considered a collaborative problem. This collaborative problem would be written as *potential complication: Nausea*.

8. The complete nursing diagnosis would be as follows: *Altered nutrition: Less than body requirements related to increased caloric needs, nausea, pain, and failure to ingest increased requirements as manifested by 3-pound weight loss and intake of 30% of meals.*

Case Study Twelve

1. The general problem areas for this client are as follows:

    a. Copious secretions
    b. Unable to communicate verbally
    c. Interrupted sleep
    d. Feels ugly
    e. Possible inadequate nutrition

2. Reclustering the data clarifies the general problem areas as follows:

Cluster One (general problem: Copious secretions)

1. Postoperative radical neck surgery and laryngectomy
2. Requires frequent oral and tracheostomy suctioning of copious secretions
3. Coughs frequently because of copious secretions
4. Unable to swallow because of tracheostomy tube

Cluster Two (general problem: Unable to communicate verbally)

1. Laryngectomy
2. Call bell for nurse
3. Pencil and pad of paper available for communication
4. Responds to questions by nodding head

Cluster Three (general problem: Interrupted sleep)

1. Surgical ICU environment
2. Requires frequent oral and tracheostomy suctioning
3. Reports being very tired

Cluster Four (general problem: Feels ugly)

1. Radical neck surgery with laryngectomy
2. Expresses disgust with his appearance
3. Cries when his wife visits; writes he is sorry he looks so horrible for her
4. Went to gym twice a week to work out before surgery
5. No friends have been in to see him

Cluster Five (general problem: Possible inadequate nutrition)

1. Cancer history
2. Radical neck surgery
3. Height 5′10″; weight 190 pounds
4. Continuous tube feedings 3000 calories per day
5. IV D_5W 125 ml per hour

3. Before making the diagnostic hypotheses, analyze the reclustered data to determine whether any additional data are needed. The additional data to collect include:

Cluster One: Copious secretions

You will want to know whether he can rinse his mouth or drink any fluids. Has anyone taught him how to suction his own mouth? Has a nurse instructed him on the importance of sitting or lying on his side rather than flat on his back? You must ask him whether he coughs or chokes, or both, every time he tries to swallow or whether there are other things that cause coughing or choking. You will ascertain that the tracheostomy cuff is inflated at the correct pressure to prevent aspiration of oral secretions.

Because of his oral surgery and sutures in his mouth, copious oral secretions, and frequent suctioning, you would also want to assess the condition of his oral mucous membranes.

Cluster Two: Unable to communicate verbally

There is already a nursing plan in place to deal with this problem. However, the nurse should evaluate whether the plan meets his current needs.

Cluster Three: Interrupted sleep

Since the major defining characteristic of a *sleep pattern disturbance* is present, you do not need any additional data.

Cluster Four: Feels ugly

Since the major defining characteristics of a *body image disturbance* are present, you do not need any additional data.

Cluster Five: Possible inadequate nutrition

To further assess his nutritional state, you will check his laboratory test results (for example, hematocrit and hemoglobin, serum albumin, or total protein level) to identify indicators of nutritional deficiency. His height and weight at this time are within normal limits.

It is important to analyze the number of calories he is receiving to determine whether they are sufficient. D_5W provides 170 kcal/L; since he is to receive 3 L/day, he will have 510 kcal/day. His tube feeding is providing 3000 kcal/day. Nutritional support required for an average adult after surgery is between 2700 and

3500 kcal/day. Therefore with the IV and the tube feeding, he is presently receiving adequate calories to meet his metabolic needs.

You are reminded about conflicting cues. Conflicting cues are items of information that may negate the validity of a particular nursing diagnosis. Because of the presence of conflicting cues (that is, no weight loss, adequate caloric intake, and ideal body weight), there is no diagnosis related to inadequate nutrition at this time. Mr. Jones may be at risk for this diagnosis if he receives chemotherapy or radiation therapy or has an infection. The nurse must monitor his changing caloric needs in relation to his caloric intake.

4. The diagnostic hypotheses for this case are as follows:

    a. *Risk for infection*
    b. *Impaired swallowing or high risk for aspiration*
    c. *Altered oral mucous membrane*
    d. *Impaired verbal communication*
    e. *Sleep pattern disturbance*
    f. *Body image disturbance*

5. After looking at the definitions and defining characteristics of each of the diagnostic hypotheses and using Lunney's[4] criteria for determining accuracy of a diagnosis, you can determine that all of these are accurate diagnoses for this case.

a. *Risk for infection* is defined by NANDA as "the state in which an individual is at increased risk for being invaded by pathogenic organisms."[3] All clients who have a surgical incision are technically at risk for infection resulting from a break in continuity of the skin, but they may not have additional risk factors that warrant making this a diagnosis. Mr. Jones is at increased risk because of the nature and amount of secretions that continuously contaminate the surgical site. The mouth is full of bacteria; under normal circumstances this is not a problem. However, surgery breaks the continuity of the oral mucosa and places the client at risk for infection. Copious secretions are an additional risk factor because they may pool in the mouth and act as a medium for infection. Oral suctioning can further increase the risk of infection if the catheter is not cleaned and stored properly. The trauma of suctioning can also further damage the oral mucosa, resulting in additional portals of entry for infection.

The other risk factor for this client is cancer. Often clients with cancer are immunosuppressed—from the disease itself or from its treatment with radiation therapy or chemotherapy—which places them at increased risk for infection. The presence of these risk factors makes this an accurate diagnosis.

b. The diagnoses of *risk for aspiration* and *impaired swallowing* reflect similar client issues. The definition of risk for aspiration is "the state in which an individual is at risk for entry of gastrointestinal secretions, oropharyngeal secretions, or solids or fluids into tracheobronchial passages."[3] The risk factors identified as defining characteristics of this diagnosis include presence of tracheostomy tube, tube feedings, impaired swallowing (coughing), and oral or neck surgery.

Impaired swallowing is defined as "the state in which an individual has decreased ability to voluntarily pass fluids and/or solids from the mouth to the stomach."[3] The major defining characteristics in this client are coughing and expressed inability to swallow because of his tracheostomy tube.

After a period of adjustment clients are usually able to swallow with a tracheostomy tube in place. The nurse will work with the client to carefully evaluate his ability to swallow with or without the cuff inflated. At this time the client has copious secretions that are not being swallowed and are causing the client to cough. Therefore the nurse's primary concern is with the risk for aspiration that is due to impaired swallowing. *Risk for aspiration* more clearly delineates the problem in caring for this client and therefore is more precise for guiding care. NOTE: In this case another nursing diagnosis (that is, *impaired swallowing*) is used as anetiology of the diagnosis.

c. *Altered oral mucous membrane* is defined as "the state in which an individual experiences disruptions in the tissue layers of the oral cavity."[3] The defining characteristics include oral pain or discomfort, coated tongue, xerostomia (dry mouth), oral lesions or ulcers, stomatitis, lack of or decreased salivation, edema, and hyperemia. This client demonstrates the following defining characteristics: Oral pain, edema, and hyperemia; there are no conflicting cues. Therefore this is an accurate diagnosis.

d. The definition of *impaired verbal communication* is "the state in which an individual experiences a decreased or absent ability to use or understand language in human interaction."[3] The major relevant defining characteristic in this client is the inability to speak because of laryngectomy. This is a highly relevant cue; thus *impaired verbal communication* is an accurate diagnosis. This is also an important diagnosis to treat early, since communication is so vitally important to every human being. Not only is communication necessary for one's safety, such as to call for help when having difficulty breathing, but it is a part of every interpersonal interaction. Inability to communicate threatens one's very existence.

e. The definition of *sleep pattern disturbance* is "a disruption of sleep time which causes discomfort or interferes with desired lifestyle."[3] Mr. Jones has two of the major defining characteristics: interrupted sleep and verbal complaints of not feeling well rested. The probable causes of his *sleep pattern disturbance* are the noisy environment of the ICU and the need for frequent suctioning.

f. *Body image disturbance* is defined as "disruption in the way one perceives one's body image."[3] The client has experienced a structural change in his face and neck, and he has communicated his sadness about his appearance to his wife. These are relevant, major defining characteristics of this diagnosis. Radical neck surgery and laryngectomy produce major structural alterations in the face. At this point in the postoperative period, Mr. Jones's face is probably swollen, which further disfigures him. A tracheostomy is compounding his adjustment. Interventions for this diagnosis will include explaining that his facial appearance will improve as the edema subsides, allowing him to express his feelings about his appearance, and gradually encouraging him to look at himself in a mirror so that he can begin to adjust to the changes in his appearance.

6. When a client has more than one accurate diagnosis, it is often necessary to prioritize the diagnoses. This helps the nurse recognize and treat the most important client problems. Setting priorities is a skill you will learn with practice. When attempting to prioritize diagnoses, it is helpful to consider the following:

a. Severity of each diagnosis
b. Potential for having a significant negative or harmful effect on the client
c. Whether the diagnosis is amenable to nursing intervention
d. Importance the client and family place on the problem
e. Long-range impact of treating (or not treating) the diagnosis
f. Role of other health-care providers in treating the same diagnoses

Three diagnoses are of equal, high priority in this case: *Risk for infection, risk for aspiration*, and *impaired communication*. In the immediate postoperative period you set your priorities to prevent infection and aspiration, since these would be life-threatening problems for the client. His inability to communicate could also be life threatening if he is not able to solicit help or communicate his need for assistance in a hurry.

7. The complete priority nursing diagnoses are as follows:

a. *Risk for infection related to extensive oral surgery, copious oral secretions, frequent suctioning, and cancer of the larynx*

b. *Risk for aspiration related to impaired swallowing, tracheostomy, and copious secretions*

c. *Impaired verbal communication related to laryngectomy as manifested by inability to speak*

1. The general problem areas that can be identified for Mrs. Crane include the following:

a. Not sleeping well, tired
b. Unhealthful diet
c. Continuing risk factors for CAD
d. Afraid of sleeping

2. Data clusters for the general problems are as follows:

a. Not sleeping well, tired
1. Awake from 8 PM to midnight tonight
2. Sleeps only for short intervals
3. Disturbed by noise, activity, and hospital routines
4. "Too tired" to ambulate or perform self-care
5. "Too tired" to meet with dietitian or attend discharge classes for CAD clients
6. "Afraid to go to sleep"
7. Nods off while talking with family
8. Reports feeling exhausted and sleepy
9. Occasionally confused

b. Unhealthy diet
1. Ate a high-calorie, high-fat diet before surgery
2. Weight 22% above the ideal
3. Has not met with dietitian for nutrition teaching ("too tired")

c. Continuing risk factors for CAD
1. Twenty-year-pack history of smoking
2. Sedentary lifestyle before now
3. High-calorie, high-fat diet history
4. Weight 22% above the ideal
5. Unaware of signs and symptoms of CAD; self-medicated for "stomach problems" before admission
6. Diagnosed CAD; post CABG surgery
7. Has not attended discharge classes for clients with CAD ("too tired")

d. Afraid of sleeping
1. "Afraid to go to sleep"

3. The following diagnostic hypotheses can be developed for Mrs. Crane:

a. *Sleep pattern disturbance*
b. *Fatigue*

c. *Altered nutrition: more than body requirements*
d. *Altered health maintenance*
e. *Fear*

4 and 5. This is a complex client situation. Mrs. Crane has a life-threatening disease and has undergone major surgery. She requires continuing nursing care to recuperate, establish a new, healthier lifestyle, and learn about her disease process. It is clear from the data presented that more than one nursing diagnosis is present for this client.

The diagnosis *sleep pattern disturbance* occurs when a "disruption of sleep time causes discomfort or interferes with desired lifestyle."[3] Defining characteristics include difficulty falling or remaining asleep, interrupted sleep, feeling tired, irritability, disorientation, lethargy, and listlessness. All the data clustered under the general problem of not sleeping well are consistent with this diagnosis.

Fatigue is "an overwhelming sustained sense of exhaustion and decreased capacity for physical and mental work."[3] The major defining characteristics are an ongoing, overwhelming lack of energy and inability to maintain usual routines. Other characteristics include emotional lability, impaired ability to concentrate, lethargy, and decreased performance. At first glance the diagnoses of *fatigue* and *sleep pattern disturbance* seem to be almost identical. The distinguishing factor is that *fatigue* is a sustained state of exhaustion, it is not relieved by rest or sleep.[11] *Fatigue* is caused by increased energy demands or decreased energy production rather than by lack of sleep. Many patients with CAD or other chronic illnesses have *fatigue*. It is quite likely that Mrs. Crane was fatigued before surgery as a result of compromised cardiac function. However, at the present time her tiredness is more closely related to interrupted, inadequate sleep than to increased energy demands and decreased energy production. Therefore the more accurate diagnosis is *sleep pattern disturbance*.

Sleep pattern disturbance is a highly accurate diagnosis in this case because a large number of cues are consistent with the defining characteristics and no cues conflict or would "disconfirm" the diagnosis. If Mrs. Crane's tiredness, lethargy, confusion, and other symptoms do not resolve with appropriate nursing interventions and the establishment of adequate sleep time and quality, the diagnosis of *fatigue* should be reconsidered.

When a person takes in nutrients in excess of metabolic requirements, the diagnosis *altered nutrition: More than body requirements* can be made.[3] The defining characteristics include weight greater than 10% above the ideal, sedentary lifestyle, dysfunctional eating pattern, and eating in response to nonhunger cues. Mrs. Crane weighs 22% above the ideal weight, has a reported high-calorie, high-fat diet, and has a sedentary lifestyle.

Although it would be helpful in planning interventions to have more data, such as when Mrs. Crane eats (that is, when frustrated or at certain times of day), where she eats (home, restaurant, or social settings), and a more specific diet history, sufficient cues are present to confirm the diagnosis on the basis of the available data. It is not entirely clear how or whether her eating habits will change following surgery. The fact that she has been "too tired" to meet with the dietitian for nutrition counseling and teaching contributes to the etiology of the diagnosis *altered nutrition: More than body requirements.*

The diagnosis *altered health maintenance* has been defined by NANDA as the "inability to identify, manage, and/or seek out help to maintain health."[3] The definition proposed by Carpenito[5] is somewhat different; it is "the state in which an individual or group experiences or is at risk of experiencing a disruption in health because of an unhealthy lifestyle or lack of knowledge to manage a condition." Both definitions imply that the individual with this diagnosis has a limited ability to maintain his or her own health because of decreased knowledge, awareness, or resources. The defining characteristics, as identified by NANDA, include lack of knowledge of basic health practices, lack of adaptive behaviors, inability to take responsibility for meeting basic health practices, lack of health-seeking behaviors, and lack of resources or support systems needed to obtain or maintain health. Demonstration of an unhealthy lifestyle (poor diet or high-risk behaviors) may also be a defining characteristic.[5,11]

Mrs. Crane has numerous risk factors related to CAD. She has not had time to incorporate a knowledge of "heart-healthy living" into her lifestyle. She did not recognize the signs of heart disease, nor did she seek treatment before her admission. She believes that she will be unable to stop smoking and is unable to use educational resources (the dietitian and the discharge classes) because of her tiredness. The presence of these cues confirm the diagnosis *altered health maintenance*, whether the NANDA or Carpenito definition is used.

The etiology for this diagnosis is only partially clear. Certainly, Mrs. Crane's lack of knowledge, preexisting health habits, and lack of sleep are related factors. It would be helpful to also assess her motivation to change her health habits, the importance of health and life to her, and the resources she has available to implement any desired lifestyle changes. Further assessment is needed to collect these data, clarify the etiology, and begin planning nursing interventions.

Fear is the final diagnostic hypothesis for Mrs. Crane. *Fear* is defined by NANDA as a "feeling of dread related to an identifiable source which the person validates."[3] The defining characteristic is the ability to identify the object of fear. Additional defining characteristics include feelings of fright or apprehension; withdrawal or avoidance; focusing on danger; decreased attention, performance, or control; and somatic findings such as shortness of breath, sweating, or increased heart rate.[5,11] Mrs. Crane has clearly stated that she is afraid to go to sleep. She has identified the situation that produces fear (sleep) and is demonstrating avoidance of that situation. It is not clear from the available data why she is afraid to go to sleep. Perhaps she is afraid that if she goes to sleep she will not wake up, or that she will become disoriented and wake up not knowing where she is. She may be afraid because she does not like to be alone and her family leaves at night when she sleeps. While the diagnosis *fear* can be confirmed based on the presenting cues, further assessment is needed to identify the cause of her fear. Once a likely cause for the client's fear has been determined, the nurse must validate this with the client to make sure it is correct etiology. From the standpoint of directing nursing care, it may be more useful to explore her fear as an etiology for the diagnosis *sleep pattern disturbance* than as a discrete diagnosis.

Both the diagnosis and the etiology would then direct nursing interventions, and the problems could be resolved together.

The nursing diagnoses that can be confirmed for Mrs. Crane are as follows:

a. *Sleep pattern disturbance related to fear, unfamiliar environment, and care routines as manifested by client report of inability to sleep, long periods of wakefulness with occasional dozing, episodes of confusion, and client report of being too tired for self-care, ambulation, and discharge teaching activities*

b. *Altered nutrition: More than body requirements related to high-fat and high-calorie diet and sedentary lifestyle as manifested by weight 22% above the ideal*

c. *Altered health maintenance related to lack of knowledge about heart-healthy living and the signs and symptoms of coronary artery disease and inability to access educational resources because of fatigue as manifested by presence of multiple risk factors for CAD, failure to seek medical treatment for symptoms of CAD, and unhealthy lifestyle*

6. The priority diagnosis for Mrs. Crane is *sleep pattern disturbance.* This is the priority both because it is the most immediate problem and because it interferes with the implementation of nursing interventions for her other diagnoses. Until Mrs. Crane sleeps and feels rested she will be unable to meet with the dietitian and attend the postoperative discharge classes. These are the interventions that will treat her *altered nutrition* and *altered health maintenance.*

Case Study Fourteen

1. The general problem areas for Mr. Lyle include the following:

a. Immobility
b. Inadequate ventilation
c. Pain
d. Possible financial need

2. Data for each of the general problem areas may be reclustered as follows:

a. Immobility
 1. Bilateral tibia and fibula fractures sustained in an MVA
 2. Legs casted after ORIF 3 days ago
 3. A history of juvenile rheumatoid arthritis
 4. Joint deformities of fingers, wrists, elbows, knees, and ankles
 5. Used two canes to walk before this accident
 6. Has started physical therapy to learn how to walk with crutches
 7. Decreased arm strength as a result of arthritis
b. Inadequate nutrition
 1. No appetite since accident
 2. Feeds himself with adapted utensils
 3. Eats 25% of his meals
 4. Height 5´6˝; weight 135 pounds
 5. Three days postoperative bilateral ORIF lower legs
c. Pain
 1. Complains of pain from the fractures
 2. Rarely asks for medication
 3. Holds on to the sides of his legs protectively
 4. States that he has learned how to live with chronic pain resulting from arthritis
 5. Three days postoperative bilateral ORIF lower legs
d. Possible financial need
 1. Unable to work outside of home because of arthritis
 2. Minimal income as self-employed jeweler

3. What additional data would be helpful to you in generating diagnostic hypotheses?

a. Immobility

You may want to know more about Mr. Lyle's earlier, as well as present, mobility. For example, what were his usual activities of daily living? How independent was he in his functioning? Does he require assistance with any activities of daily living now? This will give you useful information about both his abilities and his motivation to regain his mobility. Based on this information, you may identify one or more *self-care deficits.*

b. Inadequate nutrition

You need to identify why Mr. Lyle has no appetite. Factors that may decrease his appetite include pain, nausea resulting from the anesthetic or pain, and inactivity.

To identify the etiology of his inadequate nutrition, it would also be useful to identify foods that he likes. He may have a cultural preference for certain foods and therefore not be eating adequately because of their unavailibility.

To evaluate the appropriateness of Mr. Lyle's weight, you need to know the size of his body frame. If he has a small body frame, he is only 8% under his ideal weight. If he has a large body frame, however, he is 18% under his ideal body weight.

c. Pain

You need to obtain more data about Mr. Lyle's pain to find out whether he knows that there is a difference between the chronic pain with which he has been coping and the acute pain that he now has because of the injury and surgery. The specific medication that has been ordered to treat pain during this postoperative period is also useful information. You also need to know how he has been treating his chronic pain.

d. Possible financial need

Although you know that Mr. Lyle is unemployed outside the home, you do not know whether this presents a problem for the client or his family, since he is self-employed as a jeweler. Is his wife working? Are they meeting the financial needs of the family?

4. The diagnostic hypotheses for this client are as follows:

a. *Impaired physical mobility*
b. *Altered nutrition: Less than body requirements*
c. *Pain* and *chronic pain*
d. *Self-care deficit*
e. *Possible impaired home maintenance management*

5. Examination of the definitions and defining characteristics of each of the diagnostic hypotheses will enable you to make accurate diagnoses.

a. *Impaired physical mobility* is defined by NANDA as "a state in which the individual experiences a limitation of ability for independent physical movement."[3] The defining characteristics are an inability to purposefully move within the physical environment, including bed mobility, transfer, and ambulation; limited range of motion; decreased muscle strength, control, and/or mass; and imposed restrictions of movement, including mechanical and medical protocol. Mr. Lyle was admitted with a degree of *impaired physical mobility: Functional level 1*, based on the information that he has rheumatoid arthritis with severe joint deformities and uses two canes when walking. The functional level classification provided with this diagnosis delineates five levels. Level 1 requires the use of equipment or a device; level 3 requires help from another person and an equipment device.[3] Bilateral leg fractures with casts on his legs have compounded his immobility. He now requires assistance from others to learn how to ambulate with crutches, and he also may need assistance in performing some activities of daily living (level 3). *Impaired physical mobility* is an accurate nursing diagnosis.

b. *Altered nutrition: Less than body requirements* is defined as "the state in which an individual experiences an intake of nutrients insufficient to meet metabolic needs."[3] Mr. Lyle is not 20% or more under his ideal body weight, nor does he lose weight when eating an adequate amount. Since these major defining characteristics for *altered nutrition: Less than body requirements* are not present, this would not be an accurate diagnosis for him at this time. However, he is at *risk for altered nutrition*. The risk factors for this diagnosis are the catabolic state he is in as a result of surgery, his active physical therapy, and the presence of a chronic illness, rheumatoid arthritis. This *risk* diagnosis is accurate.

c. *Pain* is "a state in which an individual experiences and reports the presence of severe discomfort or an uncomfortable sensation."[3] Relevant defining characteristics exhibited by Mr. Lyle include communication of pain and guarding behavior. The presence of the highly relevant cue of complaint of pain coupled with the knowledge that he has had surgery 3 days earlier make this a highly accurate diagnosis.

He also has *chronic pain* that is due to rheumatoid arthritis, which should not be ignored. *Chronic pain* is "a state in which the individual experiences pain that continues for more than 6 months in duration."[3] His prior method of treatment may need to be altered or continued during this hospitalization.

d. *Self-care deficits* are specified as *feeding self-care deficit, bathing/hygiene self-care deficit, dressing/grooming self-care deficit,* and *toileting self-care deficit.* These are defined as "a state in which the individual experiences an impaired ability to perform or complete: feeding, bathing/hygiene, dressing/grooming, or toileting activities for oneself."[3] The NANDA Taxonomy cross-references this diagnosis with the Functional Level Classification used with *impaired physical mobility.* Since there are no data to suggest that this patient has a *self-care deficit,* it would be more useful in guiding nursing care—and more accurate—to use the diagnosis *impaired physical mobility,* as discussed earlier.

e. *Impaired home maintenance management* is defined as "inability to independently maintain a safe growth-promoting immediate environment."[3] The defining characteristics include the following: household members express difficulty in maintaining their home in a comfortable fashion, household members describe outstanding debts or financial crises, and family members are overtaxed. There are no data at this time to confirm this diagnosis. Perhaps you assumed that he is not able to earn enough money as a self-employed jeweler. You need more data about his financial status before you can identify a problem. However, given the client's chronic illness and minimal income, as well as this acute injury, the nurse would be correct in identifying this as a possible diagnosis. Then the nurse would need to collect additional data to confirm the diagnosis or rule it out.

6. The priority nursing diagnosis for Mr. Lyle is *impaired physical mobility: Functional level 3 related to pain, bilateral leg casts, weak arm muscles, and deformed joints as manifested by inability to walk independently.* This is a priority because it is essential to maintain Mr. Lyle's independence and to prevent the further deterioration of muscles or joints from disuse.

You may have felt that *pain* is the priority diagnosis. The rationale for not making this choice is that a diagnosis of *pain* does not have an etiology of immobility in this case (for example, related to immobility). Because *pain* is used in the prior diagnosis (*impaired physical mobility related to pain*) as an etiology, it will also be treated. However, the reverse would *not* be true. That is, his pain is not related to his immobility, and immobility would not be effectively treated by interventions used to treat his pain alone.

Case Study Fifteen

1. The general problem areas that can be identified for Ms. Jameson include the following:

    a. Undergoing treatment for chronic lymphocytic leukemia
    b. Inadequate nutrition
    c. "Very tired"
    d. Upset about her appearance

2. Data clusters for each general problem are as follows:

    a. Undergoing treatment for chronic lymphocytic leukemia
      1. Discharged from the hospital
      2. Going to the Cancer Treatment Center for chemotherapy and follow-up
      3. Ten-pound weight loss
      4. Alopecia resulting from chemotherapy

Additional data you might want to collect in this cluster would include the following:

      1. What have she and her husband been told about the disease, its treatment, and her prognosis?
      2. How has she responded to the diagnosis and its treatment?
      3. Has she experienced any additional adverse reactions to the chemotherapy?

    b. Inadequate nutrition
      1. "Not eating well since cancer diagnosis"
      2. Height 5′7″; weight 140 pounds
      3. Ten-pound weight loss before diagnosis
      4. Nausea and vomiting after chemotherapy
      5. Chemotherapy for 5 days every 6 weeks, repeated three times

Additional data you might want to collect in this cluster would include the following:

      1. Does she have an appetite or is she anorexic?
      2. How are the nausea and vomiting affecting her appetite? Nausea and vomiting are common side effects of chemotherapy and, if severe enough, can seriously compromise appetite and nutrition.
      3. The client noted that she has not eaten well since the diagnosis of cancer. It is important to find out whether this is an emotional response to her diagnosis or a physical side effect of her disease or treatment, or both.

    c. "Very tired"
      1. Feels very tired; therefore has not been able to exercise
      2. Sleeps 6 to 8 hours a night
      3. Takes one to three short naps during the day
      4. Unable to think clearly or concentrate

Additional data you might want to collect about this cluster would include the following:

      1. What are her hematocrit and hemoglobin? This information is important because chronic fatigue is one of the clinical manifestations of the disease that results from anemia.
      2. Does she experience increased fatigue after she has received a chemotherapy treatment? Many patients who are undergoing chemotherapy have identified fatigue as a frequent, significant treatment side effect. Fatigue usually is reported in the first 3 to 4 days following chemotherapy administration, becomes more pronounced at approximately 10 days after chemotherapy, and declines until the subsequent treatment.[21]

    d. Upset about her appearance
      1. Viewed herself as an attractive woman before she lost her hair
      2. States that she does not want to look at herself now that she has lost her hair
      3. Expresses concern that her husband will not love her anymore
      4. Cries when she discusses her appearance
      5. Husband very affectionate and supportive of wife
      6. Husband encourages his wife to put on her makeup as usual and to consider wearing head scarves if she would like to do that
      7. Used to work full-time and exercise aerobically every other day

3. The following diagnostic hypotheses can be developed for Ms. Jameson:

    a. *Impaired adjustment* or *fear* or *anxiety*
    b. *Altered nutrition: Less than body requirements*
    c. *Fatigue*
    d. *Body image disturbance*
    e. *Altered role performance* or *altered family processes*

4. Several diagnoses come to mind when analyzing the first cluster of data. *Impaired adjustment* is "the state in which the individual is unable to modify his/her lifestyle/behavior in a manner consistent with a change in health status."[3] The major defining characteristics are verbalization of nonacceptance of health status change and nonexistent or unsuccessful ability to be involved in problem solving or goal setting. Presently there are no data to accurately make this diagnosis. You may want to retain it as a *possible* diagnosis and continue to collect more data to either rule it in or rule it out.

The diagnosis of *fear* and *anxiety* should also be considered when analyzing the data in the general problem of undergoing treatment for chronic lymphocytic leukemia. *Fear* is defined as "feeling of dread related to an identifiable source which the person validates."[3] *Anxiety* is "a vague uneasy feeling whose source is often nonspecific or unknown to the individual."[3] A medical diagnosis of cancer may cause fear or anxiety in most people. But be careful! You always need the major defining characteristics before you make a nursing diagnosis. In this situation the major defining characteristics are not present. In obtaining additional data about the client's response to the diagnosis and its treatment, you may obtain confirming cues for one of these diagnoses. At the present time you cannot make either of these diagnoses with accuracy; however, you can treat them as *possible* diagnoses and continue to collect data.

Altered nutrition: less than body requirements is defined as "the state in which an individual experiences an intake of nutrients insufficient to meet metabolic needs."[3] Ms. Jameson does not have a body weight 20% or more under the ideal, which is one of the major defining characteristics of this diagnosis. However, she is losing weight and she is experiencing nausea and vomiting related to the chemotherapy treatments. Therefore she is at risk for experiencing this diagnosis, so you will initiate nursing interventions to reduce the nausea and vomiting and to maintain a high-protein, high-calorie diet.

Fatigue is "an overwhelming sustained sense of exhaustion and decreased capacity for physical and mental work."[3] The major defining characteristics are a verbalization of an unremitting, overwhelming lack of energy and an inability to maintain usual routines. Ms. Jameson's complaint of being "very tired," her need for extra naps during the day, and her inability to concentrate, work, or exercise are highly relevant cues that make this a very accurate nursing diagnosis.

Body image disturbance is defined as "a disruption in the way one perceives one's body image."[3] To use this diagnosis, the client must have either a verbal or a nonverbal response to an actual or perceived change in structure and/or function. Ms. Jameson is quite verbal about how the loss of her hair has affected her. The presence of this highly relevant cue makes this a very accurate nursing diagnosis.

Altered role performance is defined as "disruption in the way one perceives one's role performance."[3] The defining characteristics include a change in self-perception of role, denial of role, change in others' perception of role, conflict in roles, and change in physical capacity to resume role. In the activity/exercise pattern data indicate that Ms. Jameson is unable to work, which is consistent with one of the defining characteristics. However, in the role/relationship pattern there are no diagnostic cues that would indicate a problem. Since there is only one cue, this diagnosis would not be highly accurate. This diagnosis is also less useful in terms of guiding nursing interventions than *fatigue* is.

Altered family processes is "the state in which a family that normally functions effectively experiences a dysfunction."[3] The defining characteristics include the following: family system unable to meet physical needs of its members, family system unable to meet emotional needs of its members, and family unable to adapt to change or deal with traumatic experience constructively. This diagnosis is frequently used incorrectly if one does not pay attention to the definition. This error occurs if you assume that the diagnosis of cancer will have a negative impact on the family. While it is true that their family will undoubtedly be affected by the cancer diagnosis and Ms. Jameson's medical treatment, it cannot be assumed that their family processes will be altered. All data indicate that the family is supportive and helpful to Ms. Jameson. Therefore *altered family processes* is not an accurate diagnosis.

5. After considering the definitions and defining characteristics, you can identify the following nursing diagnoses for Ms. Jameson:

a. *Risk for altered nutrition: Less than body requirements related to nausea and vomiting*

b. *Fatigue related to effects of illness and response to chemotherapy as manifested by feeling very tired, needing extra sleep, and inability to concentrate*

c. *Body image disturbance related to alopecia and changed ability to work and exercise as manifested by inability to look at self, crying, and expressing concern about husband's response to her now*

6. In this case it is difficult to isolate one diagnosis as a priority. To identify the priority nursing diagnosis, you should ask Ms. Jameson which problem is of most concern to her. This emphasizes the client's involvement in the process. Her fatigue is most likely the most important issue in terms of physical needs because of the nature of her illness and the chemotherapy. Fatigue may also complicate her altered nutrition and her ability to cope with her changed body image.

Since no one diagnosis is of obvious higher priority than any other, if the client would like nursing assistance in treating one diagnosis first, that diagnosis would be identified as the priority. However, each identified diagnosis requires nursing intervention and should be treated.

Case Study Sixteen

1. The general problem areas for Mrs. Schwartz are as follows:

 a. Dribbling of urine
 b. Decreased fluid intake
 c. Isolating herself at home
 d. Feels bad about self
 e. Red, raw perineum

2. When the data are reclustered according to the general problem areas identified earlier, the following clusters emerge:

 a. Dribbling of urine
  1. Loses small amount of urine when lifting grandchildren, coughing, or laughing
  2. Wears perineal pad to keep from soiling clothes
  3. Restricting activities and fluid intake to decrease dribbling
  4. Feels "like a baby" when she leaks urine
  5. Is reluctant to leave home for fear of urine smell offending someone
  6. Slight odor of urine
 b. Decreased fluid intake
  1. Has limited fluid intake in attempt to decrease dribbling
  2. Complains of burning in perineal area when urinating
  3. Skin dry, prolonged tenting
  4. Mucous membranes dry
 c. Isolating herself at home
  1. Is reluctant to leave home for fear of urine smell offending someone
 d. Feels badly about self
  1. Feels "like a baby" when she leaks urine
 e. Red, irritated perineum
  1. Complains of burning in perineal area when urinating
  2. Perineum red and irritated

Notice that every identified piece of subjective or objective data is used in the reclustering. Some of the strengths noted, such as "considers herself to be in good health" and "has husband of 55 years," are important data and should be considered when planning appropriate interventions. Not all data must be used when developing the problem list. Data must be retained, however, until it becomes clear that they are not pertinent to the diagnosis/diagnoses under consideration.

3. The diagnostic hypotheses for this case include the following:

 a. *Stress incontinence*
 b. *Fluid volume deficit*
 c. *Social isolation*
 d. *Body image disturbance*
 e. *Impaired skin integrity*

4. Often, additional questions come to mind and you want to perform additional assessments to "fill in the pieces." Perhaps a critical cue was not apparent on the first round of assessment, and you need to clarify the point before you accept or reject a hypothesis. In this case, however, the cues are sufficient for you to proceed with your analysis of the proposed hypotheses.

5 and 6. At this point, none of the preceding hypotheses can be eliminated. They are all supported by the NANDA definition of the diagnostic label and have one or more of the defining characteristics necessary to select the diagnosis. Although all the diagnoses are accurate, the diagnosis of *stress incontinence* is the priority diagnosis because it is the etiology of all subsequent diagnoses.

Stress incontinence is defined as "the state in which an individual experiences a loss of urine of less than 50 ml occurring with increased abdominal pressure."[3] The major defining characteristic of reported or observed dribbling with increased abdominal pressure is present. In the case of Mrs. Schwartz the probable etiology of her stress incontinence is age-related—degenerative changes in the pelvic muscles and structural supports. Because of these changes, there is leakage of urine when intraabdominal pressure exceeds the resistant pressure of the bladder sphincter.

Once stress incontinence became a problem, Mrs. Schwartz initiated activities that caused other problems to develop. The dribbling of urine caused her to restrict her fluid intake, leading to concentrated urine and dryness of the skin and mucous membranes. The concentrated, dribbling urine was irritating to her perineum, causing redness and pain on urination. The dribbling caused Mrs. Schwartz to use a perineal pad, which further irritated the area and was a potential source of odor. The fear of odor caused her to isolate herself for fear of offending others. This case is a good illustration of a single event—stress incontinence—leading to a complex of other problems.

The other nursing diagnosis that needs immediate intervention is *impaired skin integrity. Impaired skin integrity* is defined as "a state in which the individual's skin is adversely altered."[3] The defining characteristics for this diagnosis are disruption of skin surface, destruction of skin layers, and invasion of body structures. This is a very accurate diagnosis for Mrs. Schwartz because of the number of highly relevant cues that are present in the database. The red, inflamed perineum is a source of discomfort for Mrs. Schwartz, and a definite plan for relief would be needed.

7. The priority diagnosis for this case is as follows: *Stress incontinence related to age-related changes in the pelvic muscles and structural supports as manifested by dribbling of small amounts of urine when doing activities which increase abdominal pressure.* The diagnosis of *impaired skin integrity* is of only slightly less priority. The complete nursing diagnosis for the problem would be *impaired skin integrity related to stress incontinence as manifested by red, irritated perineum.*

Although the other hypothesized diagnoses are accurate, they do not have the same priority as the two noted earlier. The priority diagnosis of *stress incontinence* is most useful in planning and implementing care for Mrs. Schwartz. Once her stress incontinence is managed (probably through a program of Kegel's exercises and practice in starting and stopping her stream when urinating), the other diagnoses will no longer be problematic and will not require nursing interventions. Because it may take some time for the stress incontinence to improve, it is important that a plan of skin care be implemented until the cause of the problem is no longer present. In this case the diagnosis and treatment of *stress incontinence* are pivotal in eliminating the other problems.

Case Study Seventeen

1. The general problems that can be identified for Mr. Steven's include the following:

a. Recent death of wife
b. Ineffective management of his diabetes
c. Change in physical and social activities since death of wife

2. Data clusters for the general problems are as follows:

a. Recent death of wife
   1. Wife killed in MVA 2 months ago
   2. Reports feeling sad and angry since wife's death
   3. Reports feeling "foggy" and having difficulty making decisions since wife's death
   4. Describes self as a "sad and lonely old man"
   5. Difficulty managing own health since wife's death
   6. Has not walked, bowled, or exercised since wife's death
b. Ineffective management of his diabetes
   1. IDDM; admitted for DKA twice in last 2 months
   2. No admissions for DKA before 2 months ago
   3. Forgets to check his blood glucose and take insulin
   4. Recent change in exercise level (decreased)
   5. Has had to assume more responsibility for checking glucose, administering insulin, and planning and preparing meals since wife's death
   6. Eats many meals outside the home
   7. Can verbalize basic knowledge of diabetic diet and care
c. Change in physical and social activities since wife's death
   1. Used to walk 2 miles every day; has not walked or exercised in 2 months
   2. Used to bowl twice a month, has not bowled in 2 months
   3. Friends invite him to go bowling but he does not feel like going
   4. Sees his children regularly
   5. Continues to attend church weekly

3. The following diagnostic hypotheses can be developed for Mr. Stevens:

a. *Dysfunctional grieving*
b. *Ineffective individual coping*
c. *Ineffective management of therapeutic regimen*
d. *Social isolation*

In addition to these nursing diagnostic hypotheses, the collaborative problem, *potential complication: Hyperglycemia,* can be identified.

4 to 6. The nursing diagnosis *dysfunctional grieving* is one of two diagnostic labels dealing with grief that are recognized by NANDA. (The other is *anticipatory grieving.*) NANDA has recently defined *dysfunctional grieving* as the "extended unsuccessful use of intellectual and emotional responses by which individuals attempt to work through the process of modifying self-concept based upon the perception of loss."[3] The defining characteristics include expressions of distress, anger, or sadness as a result of a loss; alterations in eating, sleeping, activity, or libido; and altered functioning or concentration.

One problem with the use of this diagnosis is that many of the defining characteristics may also be evident as a part of the normal grief process, not just with dysfunctional grieving. Another problem is the vagueness of the concept of an extended period of grieving. Without a more specific definition, including clarification of the meaning of the term "extended," it is difficult to use this diagnosis with confidence that it accurately reflects the client's problem.

In this case Mr. Stevens' grief is not abnormal. Remember that his wife's death was only 2 months ago and he has not yet adjusted to living without his spouse. Therefore the diagnosis *dysfunctional grieving* is inappropriate. However, the fact that he is grieving for his wife may be important as a related factor (etiology) for the other diagnostic hypotheses under consideration.

Ineffective individual coping is defined as "impairment of adaptive behaviors and problem-solving abilities of a person in meeting life's demands and roles."[3] Major defining characteristics include verbalization of inability to cope and the inability to problem solve.

Minor defining characteristics are the inability to ask for help or to meet role expectations and basic needs, alterations in societal participation, destructive behavior, inappropriate use of defense mechanisms, changes in usual communication pattern, verbal manipulation, and high rate of illness or accident. This diagnosis is often the result of a situational crisis such as the death of a family member.

Recalling the clustered data for Mr. Stevens, you will see that he has some characteristics that are consistent with this diagnosis, including ineffective problem solving, decreased participation in social activities, and an increased illness rate. He is not having problems meeting his most basic needs (food, shelter, and sleep) but is having difficulty meeting the challenges of his complex medical problem (diabetes). The diagnosis *ineffective individual coping* is a viable possibility, but his problems may be more accurately expressed by the next diagnostic hypothesis, *ineffective management of therapeutic regimen.*

Mr. Stevens' grief is compromising his ability to manage his diabetes, resulting in an increase in complications. This is consistent with the nursing diagnosis *ineffective management of therapeutic regimen.* The definition of this diagnosis is "a pattern of regulating and integrating into daily living a program for treatment of illness and the sequelae of illness that are unsatisfactory for meeting specific health goals."[3] The major defining characteristic of *ineffective management of therapeutic regimen* is making choices that are ineffective for achieving the goals of treatment or prevention. Other defining characteristics include acceleration of symptoms, verbalization of difficulty managing or regulating the disease or its treatments, or both, and not including treatment in the daily routine.

In Mr. Stevens' case a number of findings are consistent with the definition and defining characteristics of *ineffective management of therapeutic regimen.* He has had an increase in occurrences of DKA, he does not make sound decisions even though he has a basic knowledge of diabetes management, he does not regularly check his blood glucose level or administer his insulin, and he does not adhere to his recommended diet. He also verbalizes that before her death his wife assisted him in managing his treatment and diet. His grief is clearly an etiology for this diagnosis.

Ineffective management of therapeutic regimen is a highly accurate diagnosis for this client. It is more accurate than *ineffective individual coping* for two reasons: A high number of cues are consistent with the diagnosis and the diagnosis provides a clear focus for nursing care. The nursing treatment of the diagnosis *ineffective management of therapeutic reg-*

imen offers the client the chance to manage his own life and disease process and helps to avoid life-threatening complications.

The fourth diagnostic hypothesis for this client is *social isolation.* This hypothesis was made based on the client's change in social activities, his refusal of his friend's social invitations since his wife's death, and his description of himself as "lonely." The definition of this diagnosis is "aloneness experienced by the individual and perceived as imposed by others and as a negative or threatened state."[3] Major defining characteristics include absence of supportive significant others, expression of feelings of aloneness imposed by others, and feelings of rejection. Other characteristics include a sad, dull affect; inappropriate interests, lack of communication, and insecurity in public. Although this diagnosis sounds good for this client, it is not an accurate diagnosis for several reasons. Even though the client states that he is lonely, he is able to identify a support system that includes family and friends. Also, he has continued to see his children and has not socialized with his friends by his own choice, not because he is withdrawn or truly isolated. It is important to choose a diagnosis based on the closeness of fit between the diagnostic cues identified in assessment and the definition and defining characteristics for a particular diagnosis. Avoid the temptation to select a diagnosis simply because the label sounds as if it is appropriate.

This client also has a significant collaborative problem. He is having difficulty controlling his blood glucose level, and this has led to hyperglycemia and resulting DKA. This problem can be written as *potential complication: Hyperglycemia.* The nurse treats this collaborative problem in conjunction with the physician. The nursing role includes monitoring the client's blood glucose level, assessing for signs of hyperglycemia, administering the prescribed insulin, identifying complications associated with hyperglycemia, and educating the client about monitoring and managing this problem.

7. After evaluating each of the diagnostic hypotheses, it is clear that only one is accurate in this case. The accurate diagnosis is correctly written as follows: *Ineffective management of therapeutic regimen related to increased self-care responsibility, grief, and changes in lifestyle following wife's death as manifested by increase in occurrences of DKA and verbalized difficulty in managing diabetes.*

This diagnosis accurately reflects the client's priority issue—better management of his diabetes to prevent the development of potentially life-threatening complications. However, *ineffective management of therapeu-*

tic regimen does not adequately express this client's other major issue, which is his response to the loss of his wife. At present there is not an official NANDA diagnosis related to grief. As nurses, however, we know that the normal grief process evokes a multitude of psychosocial, emotional, and spiritual responses and that these responses are an appropriate focus for nursing care. It is imperative that nurses recognize grief work and support the client who is grieving.

There are two ways in which the concept of normal grief could be incorporated into this client's plan of care. First, interventions for grief can be included as part of the plan for the diagnosis *ineffective management of therapeutic regimen*. This is acceptable because grief is listed as a related factor for that diagnosis and interventions should be designed to treat each related factor.

The second method that could be used to incorporate the concept of grief into the plan of care is to make the diagnosis of grieving, even though it is not recognized by NANDA. Keep in mind that it is generally difficult to evaluate the accuracy of a diagnosis that is not recognized by NANDA because no NANDA definition or defining characteristics are available. However, nurse experts such as Gordon and Carpenito,[5,9] have developed diagnoses for common problems that have not been addressed by NANDA. These diagnoses, along with their definitions and defining characteristics, can be useful in identifying nursing diagnoses and verifying their accuracy. For the diagnosis *grieving*, Carpenito[5] provides a useful definition and list of defining characteristics that are appropriate for use in making a nursing diagnosis for this client.

Case Study Eighteen

1. The general problem areas identified for this client are as follows:

    a. Poor vision
    b. Danger of personal injury
    c. Problem acquiring and preparing food
    d. Incontinence
    e. Decreasing social interactions
    f. Poor self-image

2. When the data are reclustered according to the general problem areas just identified, the following clusters emerge:

    a. Poor vision
        1. Many bruises on arms and legs from "bumping into everything"
        2. Visual acuity 20/200 with glasses
        3. No central vision
        4. Considers health good, except for vision problem
    b. Danger of personal injury
        1. Many bruises on arms and legs from "bumping into everything"
        2. Very fearful of falling
        3. Restricting activity more and more because of fear of falling
        4. Visual acuity 20/200 with glasses
        5. No central vision
    c. Difficulty in acquiring and preparing food
        1. Having increasing difficulty preparing food because of decreased vision
        2. Afraid to walk to store to do shopping
    d. Incontinence
        1. Occasional incontinence resulting from difficulty in maneuvering in strange environments and locating toilet
    e. Decreasing social interactions
        1. Restricting activity more and more because of fear of falling
        2. Stays home almost all the time; becomes irritable when family encourages an outing
    f. Poor self-image
        1. States she "feels old and useless"
        2. Fears being a burden to family

3. The diagnostic hypotheses for this case include the following:

    a. *Sensory-perceptual alteration: Visual*
    b. *Risk for injury*
    c. *Risk for altered nutrition: Less than body requirements*
    d. *Functional incontinence*
    e. *Social isolation*
    f. *Body image disturbance or self-esteem disturbance*

4. Many of the diagnoses suggested for this case are adequately supported by cues. Additional information that might prove useful in determining accurate diagnoses could include the following:

    a. What alternatives are available to her to procure food and prepare it?
    b. What are the details on the specific events surrounding episodes of incontinence?
    c. Does she desire greater socialization?

5. Close scrutiny of the definitions and defining characteristics of the hypothesized diagnoses aids in determining the validity of the diagnoses. *Sensory-perceptual alteration: Visual* is defined as "a state in which an individual experiences a change in the amount or patterning of incoming stimuli accompanied by a diminished, exaggerated, distorted, or impaired response to such stimuli."[3] The relevant defining characteristics for this diagnosis include reported or measured change in sensory acuity and indication of body-image alteration. The related factor in this case is altered sensory perception as a result of macular degeneration. This condition is due to sclerosing of the capillaries that are responsible for providing nourishment to the macula. Without an adequate blood supply the cells responsible for vision deteriorate, and central vision is reduced. The client experiences blurry vision and reduced sensory input. In this case the defining characteristics are more helpful in directing the nursing interventions than is the label of the nursing diagnosis. The close match between the cues in the case and the definition and defining characteristics make this a highly accurate diagnosis.

Risk for injury is an extremely important nursing diagnosis for the nurse to recognize and treat. It is defined as "a state in which the individual is at risk of injury as a result of environmental conditions interacting with the individual's adaptive and defensive resources."[3] The most obvious risk factors for this case are Mrs. Harper's sensory dysfunction (poor vision and no central vision) and her perceived vulnerability to falling.

Risk for altered nutrition: Less than body requirements appears to be an appropriate diagnosis. The diagnosis of *altered nutrition: Less than body requirements* is defined as "the state in which an individual experiences an intake of nutrients insufficient to meet metabolic needs."[3] There are many defining characteristics for this diagnosis; all of them deal in some way with loss of weight and ingestion of inadequate nutrients. Although the client currently appears to be in good nutritional health, she is having difficulty preparing and acquiring food, which puts her at risk for the development of altered nutrition. The use of this diagnosis directs nursing interventions that could prevent this risk diagnosis from becoming an actual diagnosis.

The problem of incontinence must be clarified by the use of the appropriate descriptor such as stress, urge, or functional incontinence. Based on Mrs. Harper's difficulty in maneuvering in strange environments and locating the toilet, the most accurate diagnosis would be *functional incontinence. Functional incontinence* is defined as "the state in which an individual experiences an involuntary, unpredictable passage of urine."[3] This definition is broad and gives little help in making an accurate diagnosis. However, the defining characteristics and related factors for the diagnosis aid in clarifying the diagnosis. The defining characteristic for the diagnosis of *functional incontinence* is the urge to void or bladder contractions sufficiently strong to result in loss of urine before reaching an appropriate receptacle. The relevant related factor in this case is the presence of visual sensory deficit. It is clear from the data presented that the etiology of the incontinence is related to the patient's diminished vision and her occasional inability to manage her environment and reach the toilet in time. In this instance the problem is related to her interaction with the environment rather than to a physiologic bladder problem.

Social isolation is another diagnosis to be considered. *Social isolation* is defined as "aloneness experienced by the individual and perceived as imposed by others and as a negative or threatened state."[3] The only cue currently suggestive of this diagnosis is that Mrs. Harper stays at home most of the time. Data are insufficient to make a diagnosis of *social isolation*. However, it does seem appropriate to make the diagnosis of *possible social isolation*. This diagnosis would direct the nurse to gather additional information in the pattern of role/relationship to either confirm or refute this diagnosis.

The presence of cues in the general problem related to poor self-image suggests two diagnoses. *Body image disturbance* is defined as "disruption in the way one perceives one's body image."[3] There are many subjective and objective defining characteristics for this diagnosis. The characteristic of verbal or nonverbal response to actual or perceived change in structure or function, must be present to justify the diagnosis of *body image disturbance*. In this case the client has actually verbalized the change in her perception of her body. This is an accurate nursing diagnosis for Mrs. Harper.

Self-esteem disturbance also appears to be an accurate diagnosis. It is defined as "negative self-evaluation/feeling about self or self-capabilities, which may be directly or indirectly expressed."[3] Relevant defining characteristics would include self-negating verbalization and expressions of shame or guilt. This diagnosis also appears to be accurate. However, the diagnosis of *body image disturbance* appears to be the more accurate diagnosis because the change in self-image is related to a physical change in the body as opposed to a more psychological change.

6. The diagnoses that are accurate for this case include the following:

   a. *Sensory-perceptual alteration: Visual related to decreased vision secondary to macular degeneration with loss of central vision*

   b. *Risk for injury related to poor vision*

   c. *Risk for altered nutrition: Less than body requirements related to difficulty obtaining food secondary to poor vision and fear of walking to store*

   d. *Functional incontinence related to difficulty maneuvering in environment and locating toilet*

   e. *Possible social isolation related to self-imposed activity restrictions*

   f. *Body image disturbance related to incontinence, feeling old and useless, and being a burden to family*

7. The priority diagnosis for this case is *sensory-perceptual alteration: Visual related to decreased vision secondary to macular degeneration with loss of central vision as manifested by difficulty managing necessary daily activities, "bumping into things," difficulty maneuvering in strange environments, restricting activities, fear of falling, and isolation*. Although *risk for injury* is an important diagnosis, it would be managed as a result of appropriate nursing interventions for the priority diagnosis of *sensory-perceptual alteration: Visual*. When these nursing interventions are carried out, there would be no need for a diagnosis to address the specific problem of risk for injury.

If you are just beginning to learn nursing diagnosis, you probably chose *risk for injury* as the priority diagnosis. In this instance the diagnosis of *sensory-perceptual alteration: Visual* is more accurate because it is more encompassing and contains more of the cues in this case.

Case Study Nineteen

1. The general problem areas for Ms. Sanders are as follows:

    a. Frequent urination
    b. Inability to do usual activities
    c. Inadequate sleep
    d. Sadness about lifestyle and health changes
    e. Not complying with medical regimen

2. When the data are analyzed and reclustered, the following clusters emerge:

    a. Frequent urination
      1. Does not like to drink fluids because she is always in the bathroom
      2. Feels like she spends the whole day in the bathroom and her bladder always feels full
      3. Voids frequent, small amounts with occasional dribbling
      4. Takes Lasix irregularly
      5. Palpable bladder
    b. Inability to do usual activities
      1. Experiences dyspnea on exertion
      2. Has pedal edema
      3. Is orthopneic
      4. Cannot go line dancing as usual
    c. Inadequate sleep
      1. Takes frequent rests during the day
      2. Is orthopneic, requiring two pillows to sleep
    d. Sadness about lifestyle and health changes
      1. Very depressed that she is "in this condition"
      2. "If this is not going to get any better, I do not want to go on"
      3. Family reports that she seems very upset most of the time
      4. Cannot go dancing anymore
      5. Takes Elavil 100 mg per day for depression
    e. Not complying with medical regimen
      1. When she is not symptomatic, does not take her Lasix
      2. Does not like to drink fluids because she is "always in the bathroom"

3. The following diagnostic hypotheses can be identified for this client:

    a. General problem area: frequent urination
       Diagnostic hypothesis: *Altered urinary elimination*

    b. General problem area: Inability to do usual activities
       Diagnostic hypothesis: *Activity intolerance*
    c. General problem area: inadequate sleep
       Diagnostic hypothesis: *Sleep pattern disturbance*
    d. General problem area: Sadness about lifestyle and health changes
       Diagnostic hypothesis: *Impaired adjustment*
       Diagnostic hypothesis: *Ineffective denial*
       Diagnostic hypothesis: *Ineffective individual coping*
    e. General problem area: not complying with medical regimen
       Diagnostic hypothesis: *Ineffective management of therapeutic regimen*

4. *Altered urinary elimination* is defined as "the state in which the individual experiences a disturbance in urine elimination."[3] NANDA identifies six specific types of altered urinary elimination: Stress incontinence, reflex incontinence, urge incontinence, functional incontinence, total incontinence, and urinary retention. To identify the correct type of altered urinary elimination in this client, you must examine the definitions and defining characteristics of each type carefully.

All you know from the data given is that Ms. Sanders voids frequent, small amounts with occasional dribbling. Her dribbling does not occur with increased intraabdominal pressure such as coughing or sneezing (therefore discard *stress incontinence*); she is aware of bladder filling (therefore discard *reflex incontinence*); she does not report an association between an urge to void and her dribbling (therefore discard *urge incontinence*); she does not experience an involuntary, unpredictable passage of urine that is generally due to an inability to reach a bathroom in time (therefore discard *functional incontinence*); she does not experience a continuous, unpredictable loss of urine (therefore discard *total incontinence*); you do not know if she experiences incomplete emptying of the bladder (therefore retain *urinary retention* until more data are collected). *Urinary retention* is characterized by bladder distention and small, frequent voiding with occasional overflow incontinence. Since these characteristics are the ones that she demonstrates, this is the correct nursing diagnosis.

The etiology of this diagnosis is unclear. Additional information that may help you is a urinalysis. Perhaps a bladder or urinary tract infection is present and contributes to her frequency.

An "in-and-out" catheterization for residual urine would add strong data for the diagnosis of *urinary retention.* However, the cause of the retention would still be unknown. Is she receiving any medication that affects urination? She is taking Lasix, a diuretic, and Elavil, an antidepressant. Lasix could be producing the urinary frequency. In addition, one of the side effects of Elavil is urinary retention caused by its anticholinergic effects. You will want to explore the onset of the frequency and dribbling with the client: if these symptoms started after the client began taking the Elavil, there is a higher probability that retention may be due to the anticholinergic effects of the Elavil.

The definition of *activity intolerance* is a "state in which an individual has insufficient physiological or psychological energy to endure or complete required or desired daily activities."[3] Ms. Sanders demonstrates the major defining characteristics of dyspnea and inability to perform her usual activities (dancing). Therefore this is an accurate diagnosis because it is supported by highly relevant cues.

Sleep pattern disturbance is defined as "a disruption of sleep time which causes discomfort or interferes with desired life-style."[3] Ms. Sanders reports the defining characteristic of interrupted sleep resulting from difficulty in breathing when she lies down. *Sleep pattern disturbance* is an accurate diagnosis for this client and is a common finding in clients with heart failure, who may have paroxysmal nocturnal dyspnea.

Three nursing diagnoses can be considered for the fourth cluster. One, *impaired adjustment,* is "the state in which the individual is unable to modify his/her lifestyle/behavior in a manner consistent with a change in health status."[3] Ms. Sanders demonstrates the major defining characteristic for this diagnosis—a verbalization of nonacceptance of health status change and unsuccessful ability to be involved in problem solving or goal setting.

The second diagnosis to consider is *ineffective denial,* "the state of a conscious or unconscious attempt to disavow the knowledge or meaning of an event to reduce anxiety/fear to the detriment of health."[3] You have some sense that this diagnosis may be appropriate because of her general behavior of being upset and expressing that she never thought this would happen to her. You need more information to confirm this diagnosis. For example, the following questions may come to mind:

Is she self-treating her symptoms rather than taking prescribed medications?

Is she able to admit the impact of the disease on her lifestyle?

Has she delayed seeking or has she refused health care to the detriment of her health?

Until you have the answers to these questions, you cannot confirm this as an actual diagnosis.

A third diagnosis to consider is *ineffective individual coping,* which is defined as "impairment of adaptive behaviors and problem-solving abilities of a person in meeting life's demands and roles."[3] Ms. Sanders demonstrates the major defining characteristics of verbalization of inability to cope when she says "If this is not going to get any better, I do not want to go on." Using Lunney's scale for degree of accuracy of the nursing diagnosis, this diagnosis would be rated as low in accuracy because there is only one cue.[4]

The fifth cluster suggested is *ineffective management of therapeutic regimen,* which is "a pattern of regulating and integrating into daily living a program for treatment of illness and the sequelae of illness that is unsatisfactory for meeting specific health goals."[3] The major defining characteristic is that choices of daily living are ineffective for meeting the goals of a treatment or prevention program. Ms. Sanders has made choices that support the treatment program (for example, stopped dancing) and some that do not support the treatment program (for example, she stops taking her medications when she feels better). Since both confirming and refuting cues are present, this would best be considered as a *possible* diagnosis at this time. Ineffective management of therapeutic regimen can also be used as an etiology for activity intolerance.

5. The nursing diagnoses for this case are as follows:

a. *Altered urinary elimination: Urinary retention related to effects of Elavil as manifested by small, frequent voidings*

b. *Activity intolerance related to ineffective management of therapeutic regimen as manifested by dyspnea on exertion and inability to participate in usual line-dancing activities*

c. *Sleep pattern disturbance related to fragmented sleep secondary to paroxysmal nocturnal dyspnea as manifested by inability to sleep*

d. *Impaired adjustment related to unsatisfactory lifestyle changes as manifested by verbalization of inability to accept that she cannot perform usual activities*

6. No one diagnosis in this case has a life-threatening component. The nurse should work closely with the client to identify the area of most importance to her. It appears that the client is most distressed with the changes required in her life; therefore *impaired adjustment* may be the highest-priority diagnosis at this time.

Activity intolerance related to ineffective management of therapeutic regimen is also a high-priority diagnosis for the nurse to use. If Ms. Sanders would take her medications as directed, her activities probably would not result in dypsnea and she could resume her preferred lifestyle. With treatment of *impaired adjustment,* the problem with medication noncompliance may become moot.

Case Study Twenty

DISCUSSION

1. The general problem areas that can be identified for Mrs. Doyle include the following:

  a. Respiratory status
  b. GI tract function
  c. Pain
  d. Separation from infant and child, unable to breastfeed

2. Data clusters for the general problems are as follows:

  a. Respiratory status
    1. Elevated respiratory rate (26 breaths/min); pulse rate and temperature within normal limits
    2. Shallow respirations
    3. Breath sounds diminished bilaterally
    4. Refuses to take deep breaths or use IS
    5. Is afraid to take a deep breath because of pain
  b. GI tract function
    1. One day after cholecystectomy
    2. Absent bowel sounds
    3. No flatus
    4. Abdomen moderately distended and tender
    5. Nausea
    6. Reluctant to ambulate
    7. Morphine PCA pump
  c. Pain
    1. One day after cholecystectomy
    2. Reluctant to ambulate or breathe deeply because of pain
    3. Reports abdominal and incisional pain, as well as pain with deep breathing
    4. Has a morphine PCA pump
    5. Reports breast discomfort
  d. Separation from infant and child
    1. Two children ages 3 months and 3 years
    2. Is breast-feeding but has been unable to do so since surgery; reports breast discomfort
    3. "I should be home with my children, not sick in this hospital bed"
    4. "I'm afraid my baby will forget me"
    5. "I haven't been away from either of my children since they were born"
    6. "Being a good mother is the most important thing I can do"
    7. Worried that children will "think I deserted them"
    8. Worried about her mother taking care of children: "That's my job"
    9. Crying intermittently since admission

Adequate data are provided for the general problems of respiratory status and GI tract function. However, additional assessment data would be helpful in evaluating her pain and her distress over the separation from her children. Regarding her pain, it would help to know the intensity of the pain; a pain scale could be used to obtain this information. It is also important to find out how the pain changes with position, activity, time of day, and administration of analgesia. The client's use of the PCA pump should be explored—is she using it effectively? How often is she attempting to self-administer a dose? Is she in pain, despite adequate morphine administration, or is she reluctant to medicate herself? If she is not using the PCA pump, despite being in pain, why not? Is she afraid of the narcotic? Is the fact that she is breast-feeding influencing her use of the PCA pump? The nurse would also want to know what has been done to relieve the breast discomfort that is due to the client's inability to breastfeed; for example, is she using a breast pump? How often?

More data are also needed about her separation from her children. Are the children able to visit? If not, is this because of hospital rules and regulations or some other reason? Can the infant be brought in to breastfeed? Is the client able to send pumped breast milk home to the infant? Is the client able to talk to the older child by phone? Can a family member bring her a picture of the children? The collection of these additional data will help in pinpointing her problems and their causes and will also be useful in planning appropriate interventions.

3. Based on the initial data, the following diagnostic hypotheses and collaborative problems can be identified for Mrs. Doyle:

  1. *Ineffective breathing pattern*
  2. *Potential complication: Paralytic ileus*
  3. *Pain*
  4. *Interrupted breastfeeding*
  5. *Altered role performance*

4 and 5. *Ineffective breathing pattern* is "the state in which an individual's inhalation and/or exhalation pattern does not enable adequate pulmonary inflation or emptying."[3] Defining characteristics include shortness of breath, tachypnea, changes in respiratory depth, cyanosis, altered blood gases, and altered chest excursion. Pain is a common contributing factor in the development of *ineffective breathing pattern*. Multiple diagnostic cues are present in the assessment data to support this diagnosis; it has a high degree of accuracy.

Paralytic ileus is a common complication of abdominal surgery. The risk of developing a paralytic ileus is increased by immobility and may also be associated with the use of morphine sulfate, which decreases peristalsis. Mrs. Doyle is certainly at risk for the development of this problem, which would be managed collaboratively by both nursing and medicine. This would be written as *potential complications: Paralytic ileus.*

Pain is defined as "a state in which an individual experiences and reports the presence of severe discomfort or an uncomfortable sensation."[3] Defining characteristics include verbal or nonverbal communication of pain, guarding behavior, narrowed focus, distraction behaviors, facial expressions of discomfort, and altered muscle tone, as well as physiologic changes such as increased heart rate, respiratory rate, or blood pressure. Mrs. Doyle has clearly verbalized her pain, is displaying guarding behaviors (that is, refusal to take a deep breath), and an increased respiratory rate. Further assessment, as discussed in question 2, is needed to determine why the current pain relief strategies have been ineffective. *Pain* is an accurate nursing diagnosis for this client.

Although *pain* is an accurate diagnosis, it may not be necessary to address it as a distinct diagnosis, since it is also the primary etiology for another diagnosis (*ineffective breathing pattern.*) If adequate nursing interventions for pain are included in the interventions for *ineffective breathing pattern*, it is not necessary to repeat them by identifying pain as a separate diagnosis. In such a case, the nurse asks herself which diagnosis is most useful in guiding nursing care—*pain* or *ineffective breathing pattern*—and selects that diagnosis for inclusion in the plan of care. In this case the diagnosis *ineffective breathing pattern* is the most useful because it clearly reflects the client's problem and directs the nurse to the most comprehensive set of interventions.

The nursing diagnosis *interrupted breastfeeding* exists when there is "a break in the continuity of the breastfeeding process as a result of inability or inadvisability to put baby to breast for feeding."[3] The major defining characteristic is that the infant does not re-

ceive some or all feedings at the breast. Minor defining characteristics include the mother's intent to maintain lactation, separation of mother and infant, and lack of knowledge about the expression and storage of breast milk. This mother has been unable to nurse her infant because of their separation during the mother's hospitalization. Therefore this is an accurate nursing diagnosis.

The final diagnostic hypothesis for this client is *altered role performance*. The definition of *altered role performance* is "disruption in the way one perceives one's role performance."[3] Defining characteristics include a change in perception of one's role, conflict in roles, change in physical capacity to perform one's role, and change in usual patterns of responsibility. Surgery and hospitalization have forced the separation of this mother from her children, which is clearly stressful for her. She has expressed a sense of not doing her job and fearing that her children would feel abandoned or forget her. She has never before been away from her children and is still breastfeeding the youngest child, which seem to intensify her sense of not fulfilling her role as a mother. *Altered role performance* is a highly accurate diagnosis for this client.

The accurate nursing diagnoses for Mrs. Doyle are written as complete statements as follows:

1. *Ineffective breathing pattern related to pain as manifested by elevated respiratory rate, diminished breath sounds, and refusal to deep breathe or use IS*

2. *Interrupted breastfeeding related to separation of mother and infant as manifested by lack of opportunity for breastfeeding since hospitalization*

3. *Altered role performance related to illness, hospitalization, and separation from children as manifested by multiple concerns about not fulfilling parenting duties and children's care during separation*

5.   In this case setting priorities is difficult. All the diagnoses are important and can have a major impact on this client's recovery. Her physical recovery will be most closely tied to treatment of the diagnosis *ineffective breathing pattern* (which includes pain) and the *potential complication: Paralytic ileus*. The client's emotional recovery will be strongly influenced by nursing management of her *interrupted breastfeeding* and *altered role performance*. To approach this client from a holistic perspective, care must be directed to the treatment of all these diagnoses.

The most immediate priority is the management of her *ineffective breathing pattern*; the initial nursing interventions should be directed towards this diagnosis.

Interrupted breastfeeding also necessitates quick intervention to prevent complications such as diminished milk production or mastitis, as well as to decrease the discomfort of full breasts. It may not be possible to fully resolve the diagnosis of *altered role performance* during her hospital stay. However, nursing interventions to reduce the stress caused by this response to hospitalization should be instituted as soon as possible. It is even possible that reducing Mrs. Doyle's emotional pain will help decrease the physical pain she is experiencing and speed her recovery.

Case Study Twenty-One

1. The general problem areas for Mr. Sinclair are as follows:

    a. Lack of money to purchase oxygen
    b. Fluid retention
    c. Breathing problem and cough
    d. Not following prescribed diet

2. When the data are reclustered according to the general problem areas just identified, the following clusters emerge:

    a. Lack of money to purchase oxygen
      1. Unable to have oxygen refilled because of lack of money
      2. Unemployed and receiving disability pay for 2 years
      3. Low-flow oxygen prescribed for nighttime use
    b. Fluid retention
      1. Seven-pound weight gain in last 10 days
      2. Peripheral edema
      3. Enlarged liver
      4. On low-salt diet with restricted fluids
      5. Full, bounding pulse
      6. Takes diuretic each morning
      7. Has heart failure
    c. Breathing problem and cough
      1. Unable to have oxygen refilled because of lack of money
      2. Complains of dyspnea and cough
      3. Low-flow oxygen prescribed for nighttime level
      4. Has COPD, CHF, and cor pulmonale
      5. Hematocrit 59%; hemoglobin 21 g/dl
    d. Failure to follow prescribed diet
      1. Advised to follow a diet low in salt, along with restricted fluids
      2. Eats a high-salt diet

3. The diagnostic hypotheses for this case are as follows:

    a. *Altered health maintenance*
    b. *Fluid volume excess*
    c. *Ineffective management of therapeutic regimen*
    d. *Impaired gas exchange*

4. No additional data are necessary to establish the diagnoses. However, the following additional data might be helpful in identifying related factors and planning appropriate interventions.

    a. *Ineffective management of therapeutic regimen:* What does he know about a low-salt diet?
    b. *Impaired gas exchange*
      1. What is his oxygen saturation?
      2. What do his lungs sound like?

5 and 6. The definition and defining characteristics for the hypothesized diagnoses help in determining the most accurate diagnoses. *Altered health maintenance* is defined as "inability to identify, manage, and/or seek out help to maintain health."[3] Many defining characteristics would support the nurse's decision in the selection of this diagnosis. In fact, the number and diversity of the defining characteristics occasionally make this a difficult diagnosis to recognize. In the case of Mr. Sinclair, his lack of financial resources to comply with his prescribed regimen (low-flow oxygen) is the most predictive cue for the diagnosis of *altered health maintenance.*

Fluid volume excess is another nursing diagnosis that must be explored. The definition of this diagnosis is "the state in which an individual experiences increased fluid retention and edema."[3] The relevant defining characteristics include edema, weight gain, and shortness of breath; all are present in Mr. Sinclair's database. The presence of these highly relevant cues makes this a very accurate diagnosis.

On careful analysis a seeming incongruency is present in what appears to be a very straightforward nursing diagnosis. Two other defining characteristics of *fluid volume* excess are decreased hemoglobin level and decreased hematocrit. Mr. Sinclair has just the opposite finding—elevated hemoglobin level and hematocrit. Cor pulmonale leads to chronic hypoxemia, which stimulates erythropoiesis and increases the viscosity of the blood. The elevated hematocrit and hemoglobin level are consistent with cor pulmonale and different from what is usually found in fluid volume excess. In this case, despite a conflicting cue, the hypothesized diagnosis is accurate. The nurse's knowledge of the pathophysiology of cor pulmonale helps her understand the significance of the elevated hemoglobin level and hematocrit and not to consider these two findings as cues that would invalidate the diagnosis of *fluid volume deficit*.

The etiology of this diagnosis is related to the client's inability to follow the prescribed low-salt diet. Additional assessment data would clarify whether this situation was the result of lack of knowledge of the importance of this dietary restriction to the treatment of heart failure or an unwillingness on Mr. Sinclair's part to adhere to a low-salt diet. Identifying the reason for the noncompliance would be valuable in planning appropriate interventions.

Some practitioners would argue that *fluid volume excess* is seldom a nursing diagnosis. Rather, they would state that Mr. Sinclair's problem should be considered a collaborative problem. As defined earlier in this text, collaborative problems are physiologic complications for which the nurse must monitor to detect onset or changes in patient status. Often, the most definitive treatment for the problem of *fluid volume excess* is the physician-directed use of appropriate medications to relieve the edema. From this perspective, the problem would be considered a collaborative problem and labeled *potential complication: Edema*.

In this case, however, an etiology amenable to nursing intervention has been identified—failure of Mr. Sinclair to follow his prescribed low-salt diet. His edema has persisted, despite the usual medical interventions. The primary nursing intervention would be related to the low-salt diet. In addition to this primary nursing intervention, additional nursing actions such as monitoring fluid intake and output; administering meticulous skin care; frequent assessment of weight, breath sounds, and edema; and elevation of lower extremities are appropriate interventions. These interventions would be carried out, in addition to administering prescribed medications. In this instance there are specific nursing interventions for the diagnosis of *fluid volume excess* that clearly make it a nursing diagnosis. Because highly relevant cues are present, it is an accurate nursing diagnosis.

Another hypothesis that must be considered is *ineffective management of therapeutic regimen*. This diagnosis is defined as "a pattern regulating and integrating into daily living a program for treatment of illness and the sequelae of illness that is unsatisfactory for meeting specific health goals."[3] The major defining characteristic is client choices of daily living practices that are ineffective for meeting the goals of a treatment or prevention program. Although both the definition and the major defining characteristic—failure to follow a low-salt diet—are present and would make this an accurate diagnosis, it is more useful to use these cues as the etiology for the diagnosis of *fluid volume excess*.

The third hypothesized nursing diagnosis is *impaired gas exchange*. The definition of this diagnosis is "the state in which the individual experiences a decreased passage of oxygen and/or carbon dioxide between the alveoli of the lungs and the vascular system."[3] The defining characteristics include confusion, somnolence, restlessness, irritability, inability to move secretions, hypercapnia, and hypoxia. Although the oxygen saturation is not given, the diagnosis of cor pulmonale is suggestive of hypoxia. The broad etiologic (related) factor given for this diagnosis is ventilation perfusion imbalance, again implied by Mr. Sinclair's medical diagnoses. Based on these facts the diagnosis of *impaired gas exchange related to ventilation perfusion imbalance as manifested by dyspnea, hypoxia, and cough* is a possibility. However, it has been suggested that the diagnosis of *impaired gas exchange* is not helpful in determining nursing interventions.[5] When appropriate, other nursing diagnoses related to respiratory problems would be used, such as *ineffective breathing pattern* or *activity intolerance*. When the nurse continually returns to a client's medical diagnosis in attempting to determine the etiology of a nursing diagnosis, the problem is probably not a nursing diagnosis but a collaborative problem. The most accurate label for Mr. Sinclair's problem is *potential complication: Hypoxemia*.

7. In this case both *altered health maintenance* and *fluid volume excess* are accurate diagnoses and are of equal priority. The nursing interventions for the diagnosis of *altered health maintenance* would focus on assisting Mr. Sinclair to obtain the necessary resources to have his oxygen refilled. Low-flow oxygen is the primary treatment for cor pulmonale. If the cor pulmonale is stabilized, many of the problems related to excess fluid volume would improve considerably. This intervention, coupled with the interventions for *fluid volume excess*, would make a significant impact on Mr. Sinclair's health. One complete priority diagnosis for this case is *altered health maintenance related to lack of financial resources as manifested by failure to have prescribed oxygen refilled*. The other priority diagnosis is *fluid volume excess related to failure to follow prescribed low-salt diet as manifested by weight gain, peripheral edema, enlarged liver, and full, bounding pulse*.

Case Study Twenty-Two

DISCUSSION

1. The general problem areas for Ms. Hilton are as follows:

   a. Fluid loss and dehydration
   b. Weakness
   c. Absence of normal blood pressure response to activity

2. When the data are reclustered according to the general problem areas identified above, the following clusters emerge:

   a. Fluid loss and dehydration
     1. Lost 4 pounds in past week
     2. Has dry skin and mucous membranes
     3. Complains of thirst
     4. Urinating large amounts of dilute urine frequently
     5. Resting blood pressure 94/58 mm Hg
   b. Weakness
     1. Has had increasing generalized weakness over the past 4 months
   c. Absence of normal blood pressure response to activity
     1. Resting blood pressure 94/58 mm Hg
     2. Post activity blood pressure 98/72 mm Hg
     3. History of mitral stenosis

3. The diagnostic hypotheses for this client are as follows:

   a. *Fluid volume deficit*
   b. *Activity intolerance*

4. This case presents several interesting diagnostic dilemmas. The first hypothesized nursing diagnosis, *fluid volume deficit,* is relatively subtle and without an obvious etiology. When a diagnosis is recognized by appropriate defining characteristics but no obvious etiology is present, the diagnosis can be written as *fluid volume deficit related to unknown etiology.* The definition of *fluid volume deficit* is "the state in which an individual experiences vascular, cellular, or intracellular dehydration."[3] Relevant defining characteristics include change in urine output and concentration, sudden weight loss, hypotension, thirst, and dry skin and mucous membranes. None of the laboratory values used as defining characteristics, such as change in serum sodium level, were available for evaluation related to this diagnosis.

When the etiology is not apparent from the available assessment data and is written as "unknown,"

it provides obvious direction for the nurse in gathering additional assessment data to try to determine the cause of the problem. In this case the following questions that you could ask Ms. Hilton come to mind to help identify the related factor/s of the diagnosis:

   1. What has your fluid intake been?
   2. Have you made any changes in your diet to account for the weight loss?
   3. Are dry skin and mucous membranes a new or an ongoing problem?
   4. Have you had any vomiting or diarrhea recently?
   5. Are you taking any medications or home remedies?

"Unknown etiology" differs from possible in that the defining characteristics are present, but the etiology is not evident at this time. A "possible" diagnosis describes a suspected problem for which insufficient data are currently available. Both situations direct the nurse to collect additional data.

The presence of several relevant defining characteristics directs the nurse to the accurate diagnosis, even in the absence of an apparent cause. The use of "unknown etiology" is useful when you recognize the problem but do not know the cause. The complete nursing diagnosis for this problem area would be *fluid volume deficit related to unknown etiology as manifested by unexplained weight loss, dry skin and mucous membranes, thirst, and low blood pressure.*

The second interesting dilemma that this case presents is related to the scarcity of cues for the problems of weakness and absence of normal blood pressure response to activity. Alone, neither cue is sufficient to produce an accurate diagnosis. Weakness and an unusual blood pressure response are just isolated data until they are considered together. However, based on clinical experience and nursing diagnosis knowledge, the nurse should recognize that these two cues taken together support a diagnosis of *activity intolerance.* The definition for *activity intolerance* is "a state in which an individual has insufficient physiological or psychological energy to endure or complete required or desired daily activities."[3] Relevant defining characteristics include verbal report of fatigue or weakness and abnormal heart rate or blood pressure response to activity. Other defining characteristics not available currently from the database for this diagnosis include exertional discomfort or dyspnea and electrocardiographic changes.

Ms. Hilton's complaint of weakness and failure of the systolic blood pressure to respond while there was a rise of more than 15 mm Hg in the diastolic blood pressure with activity would be recognized by the experienced nurse as indicating a problem with *activity intolerance*. Do not feel bad if you missed this diagnosis. It is subtle and may require more experience than you currently have. Additional data you might want to collect to substantiate this diagnosis and make it more apparent to you are as follows:

1. Is the client dyspneic or in pain following exertion?
2. Does the electrocardiographic report (if available) indicate pathologic changes that would support this diagnosis?

The medical diagnosis of mitral stenosis plus the history of rheumatic fever are often associated with *activity intolerance* and would be additional useful information in making this diagnosis. The nursing diagnosis would be *activity intolerance related to imbalance between oxygen supply and demand*. Both *fluid volume deficit* and *activity intolerance* are accurate because the cues support both the definition and defining characteristics of the diagnosis.

5. There is also a collaborative problem in this case. Remember that collaborative problems are physiologic complications that nurses must monitor to detect onset or changes in patient status. Which collaborative problem did you recognize? The presence of thrombophlebitis always raises a red flag to the possibility of developing a life-threatening pulmonary embolus. The collaborative problem in this case that would direct specific nursing interventions is *potential complication: Pulmonary embolus.*

6. It is not apparent which of the two nursing diagnoses is the priority diagnosis. Once additional assessment data had been gathered and the etiology of the *fluid volume deficit* had been determined, *fluid volume deficit* might emerge as the priority diagnosis. This case is quite deficient in information that would normally be available for a seriously ill, hospitalized client. The provision of limited data was intentional on the part of the authors, to allow discussion of two points. First, even when the etiology of a diagnosis is not known, a nursing diagnosis can be established based on an appropriate set of defining characteristics. Second, sometimes cues that do not seem to go together and that are identified with different patient problems actually direct the selection of a diagnosis.

The complete nursing diagnosis statements for this case would be written as follows:

Fluid volume deficit related to unknown etiology as manifested by weight loss, dry skin and mucous membranes, thirst, urinating large amounts of dilute urine frequently, and low blood pressure.

Activity intolerance related to imbalance between oxygen supply and demand secondary to mitral stenosis as manifested by statement of increasing weakness and failure of systolic blood pressure to increase and diastolic increase greater than 15 mm Hg after activity.

Case Study Twenty-Three

1. The general problem areas that can be identified for this client include the following:

    a. Anorexia and inadequate diet
    b. Fatigue
    c. Illness and impending death of wife

2. Data clusters for the general problems are as follows:

    a. Anorexia and inadequate diet
       1. Not hungry for the last 3 months
       2. Eats a small breakfast, no lunch, little or no dinner; snacks throughout the day
       3. Eight-pound weight loss in 3 months
       4. Weight is 9% below the ideal
    b. Fatigue
       1. Averages 4 hours of sleep per night
       2. Has difficulty falling asleep
       3. Is kept awake by thinking of his wife's impending death
       4. Unable to nap during the day
       5. Dark circles under eyes
       6. Yawns frequently during examination
    c. Illness and impending death of wife
       1. Wife is terminally ill with ovarian cancer
       2. Wife's condition has worsened in last 3 months
       3. Has had anorexia and a change in eating pattern since his wife's condition worsened
       4. Has had a change in activity level
       5. Has had a change in sleep pattern
       6. Has a plan to utilize hospice services
       7. Verbalizes anger over wife's illness and concerns over how he will handle her illness, as it worsens, and her death
       8. Feels good that he is able to care for wife at home
       9. Reports that wife has been his best friend since the age of 16 years
      10. Reports being afraid to talk with wife about his feelings, sadness, and fears
      11. Has had a change in sexual activity and libido with wife's illness
      12. Verbalizes that his life will never be the same
      13. Identifies a number of support systems, including family members and church members

3. The following diagnostic hypotheses can be developed for Mr. Thomas:

    a. *Altered nutrition: Less than body requirements*
    b. *Fatigue*
    c. *Sleep pattern disturbance*
    d. *Anticipatory grieving*

4 and 5. The definition of *altered nutrition: Less than body requirements* is "the state in which an individual experiences an intake of nutrients insufficient to meet metabolic needs."[3] Defining characteristics include weight loss, body weight 20% or more lower than the ideal, reported inadequate food intake, aversion to eating, abdominal pain, lack of interest in food, and various clinical findings associated with poor nutrition. NANDA has not differentiated between major and minor defining characteristics for this diagnosis.

Mr. Thomas has a reported inadequate food intake, decreased appetite, and a moderate weight loss. He is not 20% or more below his ideal weight and does not display the clinical signs of inadequate nutrition (poor muscle tone, capillary fragility, pale mucous membranes, and excessive hair loss). In this case there are a relatively small number of confirming cues present and an absence of many other confirming cues. Therefore, although not incorrect, *altered nutrition: Less than body requirements* is not a highly accurate diagnosis. Since it is clear that the client has ongoing issues related to nutrition and could face nutritional problems in the future, it is best to consider this as a risk diagnosis—*risk for altered nutrition: Less than body requirements*. The stress of his wife's illness and his anticipation of her death appear to be related factors for this diagnosis.

The hypothesis of *fatigue* can be quickly eliminated from consideration by a review of its definition and defining characteristics. It is defined as "an overwhelming sustained sense of exhaustion and decreased capacity for physical and mental work."[3] The exhaustion of *fatigue* is not relieved by sleep. This client does not exhibit the major defining characteristics, which are the inability to maintain his usual routines and the verbalization of an overwhelming lack of energy. He simply says he feels tired, yet continues to work and care for his wife. Therefore this is not an accurate diagnosis.

Sleep pattern disturbance is present when a "disruption of sleep time causes discomfort or interferes with desired life-style."[3] Mr. Thomas displays two of the major defining characteristics of this diagnosis—difficulty falling asleep and not feeling well rested. He also displays several minor characteristics, including dark circles under his eyes and frequent yawning. *Sleep pattern disturbance* is an accurate diagnosis. The etiology for this diagnosis is Mr. Thomas's anticipation of his wife's death.

The third diagnostic hypothesis for this client is *anticipatory grieving*. NANDA has recently defined *anticipatory grieving* as "intellectual and emotional responses and behaviors by which individuals work through the process of modifying self-concept based on the perception of potential loss."[3] The defining characteristics include potential loss of a significant object (or person); expression of distress at potential loss; guilt, anger, or sorrow; changes in eating, sleeping, or activity habits; altered libido; and altered communication pattern. Mr. Thomas exhibits almost all of these findings. He is facing his wife's death and has verbalized his distress over this impending loss. He is angry and sad. He has had changes in his eating habits, his sleep pattern, his activity level, and his libido. He has also changed the way he communicates with his wife. *Anticipatory grieving* is a highly accurate diagnosis in this case.

6. Up to this point, you have identified three accurate diagnoses (*high risk for altered nutrition: Less than body requirements, sleep pattern disturbance,* and *anticipatory grieving*). You are now asked to select a priority diagnosis. Begin by asking yourself this question: Is there a connection between the diagnosis of *anticipatory grieving* and the other two diagnoses? In this case the illness of Mr. Thomas's wife, his anticipation of her death, and his awareness of how his life will change after her death provide a common etiology

for all three diagnoses. When multiple diagnoses are linked by a common etiology, the nurse often finds that treating one of the diagnoses leads to improvement in the other diagnoses. In this case treatment of the diagnosis *anticipatory grieving*, which is also the most highly accurate of the diagnoses, will affect all three of the diagnoses. As this client finds outlets for his grief and new ways to cope with his anticipated loss, his signs and symptoms will diminish. Since both of the other two accurate diagnoses in this case (*risk for altered nutrition: Less than body requirements* and *sleep pattern disturbance*) are essentially signs and symptoms of *anticipatory grieving*, they, too, will resolve as his *anticipatory grieving* is treated. For this reason, *anticipatory grieving* is the priority diagnosis.

It is beyond the scope of this text to address the planning stage of nursing process; however, this case study provides a good example of how assessment data that are not particularly useful in diagnosis can be quite useful in planning care. In planning care for Mr. Thomas, the nurse should reexamine the clustered cues to identify his strengths and resources. The data contain a number of these cues, including his family support, his ability to talk to his brother, his support from church members, his belief that God will help him cope with the loss of his wife, his plan to use a hospice service, and his positive self-perception that he is being a good husband and doing everything he can to care for his wife at home. These cues provide valuable information that can be used to develop individualized interventions. These nursing interventions will help Mr. Thomas identify coping mechanisms, support systems, and ways to deal with his *anticipatory grieving*.

7. The most accurate diagnosis is correctly written as follows: *Anticipatory grieving related to wife's impending death from ovarian cancer as manifested by verbalizations of sadness and anger and changes in patterns of eating, sleeping, activity, and libido.*

Case Study Twenty-Four

1. The general problem areas for Ms. Lucero are as follows:

  a. Fatigue
  b. Inadequate health practices
  c. Unremitting care responsibilities for mother
  d. Obesity
  e. Constant dull headache
  f. Inability to concentrate
  g. No social relationships

2. When the data are reclustered according to the general problem areas just identified, the following clusters emerge:

  a. Fatigue
    1. Complains of being exhausted
    2. Has no regular exercise program
    3. Has no complaints of dyspnea on exertion
    4. Is having increasing difficultly carrying out necessary daily activities
    5. Constant, dull headache
    6. Has no time or energy to pursue social relationships
    7. Has occasional inability to concentrate
  b. Inadequate health practices
    1. Has not had a Pap test for 6 years
    2. Has never had a mammogram
    3. Has no chronic illnesses
    4. Eats a high-starch, high-sugar diet
    5. Has no regular exercise program
  c. Unremitting care responsibilities
    1. Complains of overwhelming sense of fatigue
    2. Is having increasing difficulty carrying out necessary daily activities
    3. Quit work 6 years ago to care for mother full-time
    4. Has no relief from caregiving responsibilities
  d. Obesity
    1. Eats a high-starch, high-sugar diet
    2. Is 22% above the ideal body weight
    3. Has no regular exercise program
  e. Headache
    1. Complains of constant, dull headaches
  f. No social relationships
    1. Has no relief from caregiving responsibilities
    2. Complains of overwhelming sense of fatigue
    3. Quit work 6 years ago to care for mother full-time
    4. Has no time or energy to pursue social relationships

3. Many diagnostic hypotheses must be considered for this case. The most apparent diagnostic hypotheses include the following:

  a. *Fatigue and activity intolerance*
  b. *Altered health maintenance*
  c. *Risk for caregiver role strain*
  d. *Altered nutrition: More than body requirements*
  e. *Impaired home maintenance management*
  f. *Pain*
  g. *Impaired social interaction* or *social isolation* or *diversional activity deficit*

4. Additional data that could prove useful in establishing the accuracy of the hypothesized nursing diagnoses include the following:

  a. What is the quality of her sleep?
  b. Does she feel less fatigued after sleep?
  c. What alternate care situations has she used in the past?
  d. What specific daily activities are problematic for her?
  e. Were headaches a problem for her before she became the caregiver for her mother?
  f. How does she feel about her lack of social interactions?

5. As you evaluate the definitions and defining characteristics of *fatigue* and *activity intolerance,* it becomes apparent how similar these two diagnoses are. Which is the more appropriate diagnosis for this set of defining characteristics? *Fatigue* is defined as "an overwhelming sustained sense of exhaustion and decreased capacity for physical and mental work."[3] The major defining characteristics are verbalization of an unremitting, overwhelming lack of energy and inability to maintain usual routines. Minor characteristics that are relevant to this case include impaired ability to concentrate and disinterest in surroundings. *Activity intolerance* is defined as "a state in which an individual has insufficient physiological or psychological energy to endure or complete required or desired daily activities."[3] The defining characteristics include verbal report of fatigue or weakness, abnormal heart rate or blood pressure in response to activity, exertional discomfort or dyspnea, and electrocardiographic changes reflecting arrhythmias or ischemia.

Both diagnoses have definitions that are appropriate for this problem. As the defining characteristics are examined, however, the physiologic overtones inherent in the diagnosis of *activity intolerance* become obvious. Also, the related factors help make apparent the more accurate and specific nursing diagnosis. The relevant related factors for *fatigue* are overwhelming psychological or emotional demands and excessive social and/or role demands. Related factors for *activity intolerance*, again, indicate a greater physiologic basis in such factors as bedrest or immobility; generalized weakness; sedentary lifestyle; and imbalance between oxygen supply and demand. On close examination of the cues clustered under *fatigue*, it becomes clear that *fatigue* is the more accurate diagnosis for this problem.

Altered health maintenance is another nursing diagnosis that seems appropriate for this case. *Altered health maintenance* is defined as "inability to identify, manage, and/or seek out help to maintain health."[3] The relevant defining characteristics include reported or observed inability to take responsibility for meeting basic health practices in any functional health pattern and history of lack of health-seeking behavior. It is not yet known whether another important defining characteristic for this diagnosis, demonstrated lack of knowledge regarding basic health practices, is relevant in this case. Ms. Lucero's failure to have an annual Pap test or baseline mammogram, plus her unhealthful diet, obesity, and lack of regular exercise, all support the accuracy of this diagnosis. Lack of knowledge regarding health practices or the constant attention to the needs of her mother and the consequent exhaustion could be etiologies for this diagnosis.

Another diagnosis that seems fairly obvious from the cues presented is *risk for caregiver role strain*. It is tempting to assign the actual diagnosis of *caregiver role strain*, but evaluation of the definitions and defining characteristics make it clear that it is more accurate as a *risk* diagnosis. *Risk for caregiver role strain* is defined as follows: "a caregiver is vulnerable for felt difficulty in performing family caregiver role."[3] There are many risk factors identified for this diagnosis related to pathophysiologic, development, psychological, and situational factors. The most relevant ones for this case include the following: illness severity of the care receiver (advanced Alzheimer's disease); caregiver is female (daughter); care receiver exhibits deviant, bizarre behavior (possible problem that is due to care receiver's diagnosis); caregiver isolation (has no time or energy to pursue social relations); lack of respite and recreation for caregiver (has no relief from caregiving responsibilities); caregiver not developmentally ready for caregiver role (quit work to care for mother); caregiver health impairment (overwhelming exhaustion at age 51 years); and amount of caregiving tasks (total care on 24-hour basis and not able to carry out necessary daily activities).

The actual diagnosis of *caregiver role strain*, is defined as "a caregiver's felt difficulty in performing the family caregiver role." Many defining characteristics are listed for this diagnosis. Many of these characteristics and risk factors are the same for both diagnoses. At this point, however, the caregiver has not verbalized any difficulty in performing the caregiving functions, which is a necessary characteristic for the diagnosis. Only risk characteristics are currently present. Further discussion with Ms. Lucero regarding her perceived ability to manage the caregiving tasks for her mother may provide the data needed to assign the actual diagnosis. Until such validating data are available, the diagnosis of *risk for caregiver role strain* is the more accurate diagnosis.

Impaired home maintenance management also appears to be an appropriate diagnosis for this case. It is defined as "inability to independently maintain a safe growth-promoting immediate environment."[3] There are many critical defining characteristics for this diagnosis, such as household members expressing difficulty in maintaining their home in a comfortable fashion, household members describing outstanding debts or financial crises, disorderly surroundings, and overtaxed family members. Although not all of the many critical defining characteristics for this diagnosis are present, at least two (increasing difficulty carrying out necessary daily activities and overtaxed family member) are present. Although this may not be a priority diagnosis at this time, it is an accurate diagnosis.

Pain is also an accurate diagnosis because it meets the criterion of the definition, "a state in which an individual experiences and reports the presence of severe discomfort or an uncomfortable sensation."[3] Ms. Lucero complains of a constant, dull headache, which meets the requirement of the defining characteristic of communication of pain descriptors. Again, although this is an accurate diagnosis, it is probably not a priority diagnosis in view of the total situation. Additional data related to a history of headaches before the increase in caregiving responsibilities would be important in deciding about the relevance of this cue. If headaches were not a problem before the client began taking on the caregiving responsibility for her mother, initiation of appropriate nursing interventions related to *fatigue* and *risk for caregiver role strain* would probably resolve the problem of the dull headaches. The constant, dull headache is better used as a defining characteristic for these two nursing diagnoses rather than as a defining characteristic for the separate nursing diagnosis of *pain*.

The cues clustered in the general problem area related to lack of social relationships are difficult to label. Three nursing diagnoses can be considered for this set of cues: *impaired social interaction, social isolation,* and *diversional activity deficit. Impaired social interaction* is defined as "the state in which an individual participates in an insufficient or excessive quantity or ineffective quality of social exchange."[3] The major defining characteristics are verbalized or observed discomfort in social situations; verbalized or observed inability to receive or communicate a satisfying sense of belonging, caring, interest, or shared history; observed use of unsuccessful social interaction behaviors; and dysfunctional interaction with peers, family, or others. None of the cues about Ms. Lucero's social relationships that have been presented in this case are consistent with the critical cues for the diagnosis of *impaired social interaction.* Therefore this diagnosis is inaccurate and to pursue it would be incorrect.

Social isolation is another nursing diagnosis that appears to be appropriate for this case. It is defined as "aloneness experienced by the individual and perceived as imposed by others and as a negative or threatened state."[3] Two critical subjective defining characteristics for this diagnosis—expresses feelings of aloneness imposed by others and expresses feelings of rejection—are not present in the database. One critical defining characteristic, absence of supportive significant other/s, is present. It appears that additional data are needed to make the actual diagnosis of *social isolation.* However, based on the cues present and the nurse's knowledge of the course of Alzheimer's disease and similar care situations, the diagnosis of *possible social isolation* is appropriate and would direct the collection of additional data to confirm or refute this diagnosis.

Diversional activity deficit is also a diagnosis worth considering for this case. It is defined as "the state in which an individual experiences decreased stimulation from or interest or engagement in recreational or leisure activities."[3] The defining characteristics include the client's statements about boredom, such as "wish there was something to do" or "to read" and about usual hobbies that cannot be undertaken in the hospital. It is obvious from examination of the defining characteristics that this is not an appropriate diagnosis for this case. The client has not expressed any problem

with boredom. In fact, her problem is not having enough time to do what needs to be done. If you considered this diagnosis, it may be a situation of imposing your own values on a client. One may think a person would be bored having nothing to do but care for an ill mother. In fact, this is probably not the situation for this client.

6. The accurate diagnoses that remain after careful consideration of all hypotheses include the following:

   a. *Fatigue related to unremitting care responsibilities without respite*
   b. *Altered health maintenance related to constant needs of mother and state of exhaustion*
   c. *Risk for caregiver role strain related to unremitting care responsibilities of mother with Alzheimer's disease*
   d. *Impaired home maintenance management related to constant needs of mother and state of exhaustion*
   e. *Possible social isolation related to inability to pursue social activities, lack of support, and state of exhaustion*

7. There is probably not one clear-cut priority diagnosis for this case. Both *fatigue* and *risk for caregiver role strain* are very important diagnoses and require immediate nursing interventions. *Altered health maintenance* is also an important diagnosis but does not carry the urgency of the other two priority diagnoses. Once the situation has stabilized, the nurse would plan interventions appropriate for the diagnosis of *altered health maintenance.*

The complete nursing diagnoses for the two priority diagnoses would be written as follows:

1. *Fatigue related to unremitting care responsibilities without respite as manifested by overwhelming sense of exhaustion, increasing difficulty carrying out necessary daily activities, occasional inability to concentrate, no energy to pursue social relationships, and constant, dull headache*

2. *Risk for caregiver role strain related to unremitting care responsibilities of mother with Alzheimer's disease*

Case Study Twenty-Five

PART ONE

1. A number of factors increase the complexity of this case. The severity of the client's illness, along with his uncertain outcome, is one factor. In addition, there are a multitude of psychosocial issues associated with a diagnosis of cancer. Another factor is that the treatment for Hodgkin's disease is prolonged and affects not just the client but the entire family. The disease and its treatment have a profound effect on both the client's and the family's lives and futures, including their home life, work life, and ability to conceive.

If you are a nursing student you may not yet have acquired the depth of clinical knowledge and experience needed for assessment, diagnosis, and treatment of Mr. Winter and his family. If this is the case, use a medical-surgical textbook as a reference as you work through this case study. You will need a basic understanding of Hodgkin's disease and its treatment, as well as an understanding of the psychosocial and family issues associated with the treatment of cancer before you proceed.

2. This client interaction takes place in the oncology clinic. There are two purposes for the visit. One is to assess Mr. Winter's ability to care for his central-line catheter. The second purpose is to administer a dose of chemotherapy; this should include an evaluation of his response to the previous dose. Another important component to consider when looking at the context of the visit is that the client's wife has accompanied him to this appointment. This provides an opportunity to observe the couple's interactions, to assess their mutual and individual support systems, and to identify the stressors and concerns of both partners.

The nurse in this case has collected a large amount of data. Many of the data are signs and symptoms of Hodgkin's disease. As the nurse, you must have a basic understanding of this disease process to identify findings that are due to the pathophysiologic features associated with Hodgkin's disease. These findings include fatigue, weight loss, fever, difficulty in swallowing, shortness of breath, and nonproductive cough. These symptoms primarily support the client's medical diagnosis; they may also help in the identification of nursing diagnoses.

Although many data are available, the nurse in this case has failed to collect some data that are crucial to one of the stated purposes of the visit—to assess the client's ability to care for his central line. There is no evidence that the nurse has asked him to verbalize his understanding of the care of his atrial line or to demonstrate specific care techniques. It may be possible for the nurse to make diagnoses based on the data that have been obtained; however, data are inadequate to make conclusions about his self-care techniques. In collecting data it is always important to remember the context of the client situation, including the intended purpose of the client-nurse interaction. Without such consideration the opportunity to collect information about important client problems may be missed.

ADD THE FOLLOWING DATA TO THE DATABASE FOR THIS CLIENT

Health perception/health management pattern

1. When asked to demonstrate the procedure for flushing his atrial catheter the client:
   a. Does not wash his hands until reminded by the nurse
   b. Cleanses the catheter port with alcohol for 10 seconds in preparation for flushing
   c. Blows on the alcohol to get it to dry quickly
2. States that "I really don't remember everything they taught me about doing this"
3. Is unable to verbalize any of the signs and symptoms that would indicate a complication associated with central lines

Role/relationship pattern

1. Wife expresses that she doesn't want to learn how to do his central-line care because she already feels she is doing more than she can between work, home, and caring for her husband and child
2. Wife states that "he can't accept the fact that he has cancer and will probably die. He refuses to help me plan for a future without him, he just thinks he'll get better with chemotherapy and some hocus pocus meditation stuff. I don't want to upset him, so I just don't talk about it at all anymore"
3. Wife states, "I'm trying to protect him from any more stress, so I haven't told him that I've used up just about all of my paid time off and may lose my job if I take any more time off. I'm now responsible for working out everything for this family alone—I just don't know if I can keep this up"

Return to critical thinking questions on p. 124.

Case Study Twenty-Five

PART TWO

3. A number of general problem areas can be identified for Mr. Winter. They are listed along with the reclustered data, as follows:

  a. Appetite and nutrition issues
   1. Twenty-pound weight loss before diagnosis
   2. Currently receiving chemotherapy for stage III(B) Hodgkin's disease
   3. Four-pound weight loss since first dose of chemotherapy
   4. Nausea and vomiting for 2 days following first dose of chemotherapy
   5. Decreased appetite following chemotherapy
   6. Difficulty in swallowing
  b. Change in energy/activity level
   1. Reports tiredness and weakness
   2. Has shortness of breath with activity and at rest
   3. Able to perform activities of daily living
   4. Hemoglobin 10 g/dl; hematocrit 30%
   5. Unable to work for several weeks because of fatigue, weakness, and shortness of breath
   6. Elevation in heart rate and respiratory rate with activity
  c. Central-line care
   1. Did not wash hands before performing line care
   2. Used alcohol to clean catheter port
   3. Allowed alcohol to dry for 10 seconds
   4. Blows on alcohol to speed up drying
   5. Unable to verbalize signs and symptoms of complications associated with central lines
   6. States that he isn't quite used to caring for his central line yet
   7. Would like his wife to learn how to care for his central line; wife does not want to learn this care
  d. Sexual concerns
   1. Reports a change in libido and sexual activity as a result of fatigue, weakness, and shortness of breath
   2. States that his change in sexual activity is "the worst part of this whole thing"
  e. Changes in self-perception and role
   1. Not able to work; on medical leave of absence
   2. States, "I feel like I'm not being a very good husband or father lately"
   3. Decreased libido and sexual activity
   4. Concerned about future fertility

  f. Effects of illness on wife and relationship
   1. Wife works full-time outside the home
   2. States, "I wish my wife would let me do more things for myself instead of babying me so much"
   3. Feels that wife is always fussing or worrying about everything since his diagnosis
   4. Wants wife to learn central-line care
   5. Wife does not want to learn central-line care
   6. States that wife is more worried about illness than he is
   7. Wife feels she is doing more than she can between work, home, and caring for her husband and child
   8. Wife states, "I'm now responsible for working out everything for this family alone—I just don't know if I can keep this up"
   9. Wife states that "he can't accept the fact that he has cancer and will probably die. He refuses to help me plan for a future without him"
   10. Wife says nontraditional healing methods are silly and a waste of time
   11. Wife is trying to protect him from stress; this has led to her not sharing information about her possible loss of job and not talking to him to avoid upsetting him.

4. The following diagnostic hypotheses can be proposed:

  a. Appetite and nutrition issues
   1. *Altered nutrition: Less than body requirements*
   2. *Impaired swallowing*
  b. Change in energy/activity level
   1. *Fatigue*
   2. *Activity intolerance*
  c. Central-line care
   1. *Risk for infection*
  d. Sexual concerns
   1. *Altered sexuality pattern*
  e. Change in role/self-perception
   1. *Altered role performance*
   2. *Self-esteem disturbance*
  f. Effects on wife and relationship
   1. *Ineffective family coping: Compromised*
   2. *Altered family processes*
   3. *Caregiver role strain (client's wife)*

5. As you can see, many diagnostic hypotheses can be generated from the data provided in this case. This is not unusual in a complex case that involves many physiologic, psychological, and social issues. Let's examine each diagnostic hypothesis for accuracy.

Altered nutrition: Less than body requirements is not an accurate diagnosis in this case. Mr. Winter's weight is within the normal range for his height, despite his illness and treatment-associated weight loss. He may, however, be considered *at risk for altered nutrition: Less than body requirements,* since his nausea and anorexia may lead to continued weight loss.

Impaired swallowing cannot be confirmed, nor can it be entirely ruled out, as a diagnosis for Mr. Winter. He has reported some difficulty in swallowing. This is a common finding when a client has mediastinal lymph node involvement associated with Hodgkin's disease. It is not clear from the data given just how much difficulty in swallowing Mr. Winter has and whether it truly affects his ability to pass fluids or solids from his mouth to his stomach. The major defining characteristic for *impaired swallowing* is the observed evidence of difficulty in swallowing, including stasis of food in the mouth, coughing, or choking. Aspiration of food or fluids is a minor characteristic. With the data currently available, *impaired swallowing* is only a possible diagnosis, indicating that additional assessment is needed before the diagnosis can be confirmed.

Fatigue is clearly an accurate diagnosis in this case and a common finding in cancer patients. Mr. Winter exhibits the major defining characteristics of verbalized unremitting, overwhelming lack of energy and the inability to maintain usual routines. He also demonstrates some of the minor defining characteristics (lethargy and decreased libido). There are also assessment data to support the diagnosis of *activity intolerance.* The major defining characteristic for this diagnosis is a verbal report of fatigue and weakness. In addition, he has the defining characteristic of dyspnea on exertion. His low hemoglobin and hematocrit levels indicate a decreased oxygen-carrying capacity, which is a related factor for the diagnosis of *activity intolerance.*

The diagnoses of *fatigue* and *activity intolerance* are similar and may have similar interventions; therefore it is not necessary to use both diagnoses in planning care. Because the diagnosis of *activity intolerance* incorporates both the concept of fatigue and the broader issue of his inability to tolerate certain activities, it is the more useful of the two diagnoses in planning nursing care for this client.

Risk for infection is also an accurate diagnosis in this case. Mr. Winter displays multiple risk factors for infection, including the presence of an indwelling central-line catheter, decreased hemoglobin level, chronic disease (cancer), chemotherapy, and a lack of knowledge about how to avoid contamination of his central line.

Knowledge deficit is defined by NANDA as an "absence or deficiency of cognitive information related to a specific topic."[3] The defining characteristics include inaccurate follow-through on instructions, inaccurate performance, and verbalization of the problem. Because this diagnosis has such a broad definition and broad defining characteristics, it is often not very useful in guiding nursing care. A better approach is to examine the client's response to a knowledge deficit, that is, to ask what will happen to this client without an adequate knowledge base. When used in this fashion, knowledge deficit becomes a related factor or an etiology for a client problem rather than a problem in and of itself, for example, *risk for infection related to knowledge deficit of central-line care.* This diagnostic statement reflects the fact that Mr. Winter's lack of knowledge about his central-line care places him at risk for development of an infection. This provides clear direction for nursing care.

Altered sexuality pattern is also an accurate diagnosis for Mr. Winter and can be considered both as a distinct problem and as a component of his change in role/self-perception. Mr. Winter has verbalized his concern about the decrease in his libido and change in his sexual activity. He has stated that this is "the worst part of this whole thing." Assessment data are adequate to confirm *altered sexuality pattern* as an accurate nursing diagnosis.

The accuracy of the diagnosis *altered role performance* is supported by a number of cues. Mr. Winter has expressed that he feels he is not being a very good father and husband because of his illness. He no longer is physically able to perform his work role or to maintain his previous level of sexual activity. His wife also perceives that he is no longer able to perform his family role and feels that she must compensate. These findings are consistent with the defining characteristics for *altered role performance.* The diagnosis of *self-esteem disturbance* may occur in response to a change in role performance. However, few of the defining characteristics for *self-esteem disturbance* are present in Mr. Winter. Although he does express negative verbalizations about himself, these are few. He does not express shame or guilt, only that he wishes he could do more for his family. He does not reject possible feedback or exaggerate negative feedback, nor does he deny problems or project blame on others. Therefore *self-esteem disturbance* is not an accurate diagnosis in this case.

Two family diagnoses were proposed in this case: *ineffective family coping* and *altered family process. Ineffective family coping: Compromised* reflects a situation in which a normally supportive significant other (in this case Mr. Winter's wife, Victoria) provides "insufficient, ineffective or compromised support, comfort, assistance, or encouragement"[3] needed by a client to manage a health problem. To make this diagnosis, both the client and the significant other must be included in the nurse's assessment. Mr. Winter and his wife display a number of the defining characteristics of this diagnosis, including the client's perception that his wife is more concerned about his illness than he is; is babying, fussing, and worrying over him; and won't let him do even the things that he could. Another finding consistent with this diagnosis is that Victoria Jacobsen is focused on her own reactions to her husband's illness, including her fear that he will die and her need to provide care for him while still working and caring for her child and home. She also does not want to learn central-line care at this time because she is already overwhelmed by her responsibilities. Her overprotectiveness and change in communication pattern with her husband provide additional supporting data. *Ineffective family coping: Compromised* is a highly accurate nursing diagnosis.

The second diagnostic hypothesis related to family issues, *altered family processes,* is not an accurate diagnosis. The defining characteristics for this diagnosis describe a dysfunctional family unable to meet the physical, emotional, and spiritual needs of the family members. In addition, this diagnosis reflects a lack of respect among family members and a family that cannot seek help or make effective decisions.[3] In essence, *altered family processes* describes a family lacking the resources to adjust to a crisis. This is not an accurate diagnosis for this family, who may be having difficulty adjusting to the client's illness but still have strengths and resources and are, meeting at least the basic needs of each family member.

The client's wife in this case demonstrates some of the defining characteristics of *caregiver role strain.* These characteristics include lack of resources to provide the needed care, worry about her own emotional state, and her perception that she does not have the ability to both provide care and continue with the other responsibilities in her life. At this point it would be accurate to write this as an actual diagnosis. Additional data collection would increase its accuracy by identifying additional diagnostic cues.

To review, several accurate diagnoses have been identified in this case, including the following:

a. *Risk for altered nutrition: Less than body requirements related to nausea, vomiting, anorexia, and effects of disease process as manifested by 24-pound weight loss*

b. *Activity intolerance related to fatigue, weakness, and anemia as manifested by shortness of breath with activity, inability to work, and decreased sexual activity*

c. *Altered sexuality pattern related to fatigue, weakness, nausea, and shortness of breath as manifested by client report of distress over changes in libido and sexual activity*

d. *Risk for infection related to knowledge deficit of central-line catheter care, the effects of Hodgkin's disease, chemotherapy, and suboptimal nutrition*

e. *Altered role performance related to the effects of Hodgkin's disease and its treatment as manifested by client's concern over changes in ability to perform home, family, and work responsibilities*

f. *Ineffective family coping: compromised related to stress of husband's illness and strained resources as manifested by ineffective communication patterns, perceived inadequate support by both partners, and conflicting needs and values*

g. *Caregiver role strain (client's wife) related to severity and uncertain outcome of spouse's illness and responsibility for husband's care at home as manifested by wife's concerns about own ability to continue providing care for client and difficulty coordinating home and work responsibilities*

6. Question 6 asks you to examine your own beliefs and biases to determine whether they may have influenced your diagnostic reasoning in this case. Each of us have certain beliefs, preconceptions, biases, likes, and dislikes that can influence our response to a client or a clinical situation. These same factors can also hinder our ability to clearly perform assessment, diagnosis, and treatment of clients. The professional role does not demand that we give up our deeply held beliefs, only that we identify and examine them to be sure that they do not prevent us from delivering openminded, nonjudgmental, supportive client care.

To answer question 6, examine your feelings about having cancer, the use of alternative therapies (such as therapeutic touch, meditation, visualization, and herbal therapy), and the importance of organized religion in a person's life.

A nurse who harbors a personal belief that cancer is always a fatal illness, or who does not believe in the use of nontraditional therapies as adjunct treatments, may have proposed the diagnoses *hopelessness, powerlessness,* or *ineffective denial* in this case. However, none of these are accurate diagnoses for Mr. Winter. He is in fact quite hopeful about his chances for recovery, and there are no data to support the diagnosis of *hopelessness*. Although cure rates for clients with stage III(B) Hodgkin's disease are not as good as for clients with stage I, II, or III(A) disease, it is still possible for a cure to be achieved. Mr. Winter's optimism is a strength as he enters treatment.

This client also does not present data to support a diagnosis of *powerlessness*. In fact, he expresses the belief that he must actively help in making himself well. He has also begun to use visualization as an aid in his recovery and would like to try other nontraditional healing methods. Even if the nurse does not personally hold these beliefs, she must support the client in a way that empowers him to participate in his own recovery.

A diagnosis of *ineffective denial* is also inaccurate. If Mr. Winter had *ineffective denial*, he would use denial of the facts of his illness to decrease his anxiety or fear. Diagnostic cues that might be seen in his assessment data would include not seeking treatment, not keeping chemotherapy appointments, and not acknowledging the seriousness of his illness. In fact, many disconfirming cues are present in this database. The client verbalizes an understanding of his illness, treatment, and prognosis. He has demonstrated follow-through on all of his prescribed therapy. These findings are inconsistent with a diagnosis of *ineffective denial*. When nurses make inaccurate diagnoses such as these, it is often because they are placing themselves in the client's situation and expressing their own fears and concerns.

Another example of personal bias interfering with making an accurate nursing diagnosis would be the use of the diagnosis *spiritual distress* for Mr. Winter. Although Mr. Winter does not attend church or belong to an organized religion, there are no cues to support that he is having distress related to his spiritual or religious beliefs. A nurse who makes the diagnosis of *spiritual distress* in this case is probably expressing a personal judgment about a client not having a religion or church affiliation. Transferring one's own beliefs or values to a client can be a major source of diagnostic error.

7. Now that the accurate diagnoses for Mr. Winter have been identified, the nurse must set priorities. In a complex case such as this one, while all the accurate diagnoses are important in planning nursing care, some carry a higher priority than others.

In setting priorities for Mr. Winter, it is helpful to start by examining each diagnosis and identifying those which could have the most severe consequences if left untreated. These consequences may be either physiologic or emotional and psychological.

In this case the diagnosis *risk for infection* represents the greatest physiologic threat to the client. It is clearly a problem that can cause life-threatening complications. In the case of Mr. Winter several factors place him at particularly high risk for development of an infection. These risk factors include the presence of an indwelling central catheter, his incorrect techniques of caring for his catheter, his underlying disease process, and the debilitating effects of chemotherapy. The development of sepsis could be life threatening for this client. Therefore this has the highest priority of all the identified nursing diagnoses.

The other diagnoses that should be addressed as priorities are *ineffective family coping: Compromised* and *altered sexuality pattern*. *Ineffective family coping: compromised* is a priority because it threatens the client's ability to effectively cope with his illness and treatment and, if left untreated, could threaten the ability of this family to survive the stress of Mr. Winter's illness. This diagnosis is amenable to nursing management. The nurse can help both the client and his wife identify their own stressors, communication styles, and needs. Nursing care can help improve communication, increase the knowledge base of both Mr. Winter and his wife, and identify new coping mechanisms and new resources that can help them effectively manage the stress their family is experiencing.

Altered sexuality pattern is the third priority because Mr. Winter has identified it as a major concern of his. It is important to involve the client in the identification of priorities and to help resolve client-identified priority issues, even if they are not obvious threats or immediate physiologic priorities.

8. The priority diagnoses are written as follows:

a. *Risk for infection related to knowledge deficit of central-line catheter care, the effects of Hodgkin's disease, chemotherapy, and suboptimal nutrition*

b. *Ineffective family coping: Compromised related to stress of husband's illness and strained resources as manifested by ineffective communication patterns, perceived inadequate support by both partners, and conflicting needs and values*

c. *Altered sexuality pattern related to fatigue, weakness, nausea, and shortness of breath as manifested by client reports of distress over changes in libido and sexual activity*

Case Study Twenty-Six

PART ONE

1. The general problem areas identified for this client include the following:

a. Uncontrolled diabetes mellitus
b. Unhealthful lifestyle
c. Draining lesion on foot
d. Underweight
e. Dulled affect and movements
f. Poor grooming and hygiene
g. Poor vision without glasses
h. Appears defeated
i. No known sources of support
j. Loss of faith in a higher power

2. The problem areas that should be considered at this time include the following:

a. Uncontrolled diabetes mellitus. The nursing student recognizes the danger of the very high glucose level and wants to pursue this major health issue.

b. Unhealthful lifestyle. The most immediate problem related to his unhealthful lifestyle is his low body temperature as a result of cold exposure and inadequate clothing. At this time the nurse will not attempt to plan for other lifestyle problems such as grooming, hygiene, and dental care.

c. Draining lesion of foot. Although the definitive treatment for this serious lesion is not within the scope of nursing practice, the student nurse feels compelled to at least bathe the wound and cover it with a clean dressing. This is a situation in which the critically thinking nurse remains nursing focused. She recognizes that it is not within her scope of practice to directly treat the lesion. However, avoidance of further irritation or contamination of the wound is a nursing focus and is an appropriate area for nursing intervention.

d. Appears defeated. Although this problem does not have physiologic urgency, the client's present emotional state is affecting the student's ability to gather information important to accurate diagnosing. Because the student wants to provide the best care possible to this client, despite her personal feelings, she does not want to eliminate consideration of the problem at this time.

Although the other identified problems are important, planning for their resolution is not urgent and

could be deferred. For instance, obtaining new glasses for this gentleman is important and could perhaps be accomplished by a phone call to the Lion's Club Eyeglass Bank. However, the Bank is not open at this hour, and other problems are more pressing. Ultimately, adequate vision would be important for this man for such important tasks as monitoring his glucose levels, reading a phone book and dialing a phone, writing a letter or filling out a job application, reading health education literature, or simply reading for pleasure to maintain contact with everyday life.

Now that the student has narrowed the problem areas to a more manageable number, she proceeds with the next step of this process.

3. The appropriate data for the problem areas would be reclustered as follows:

a. Uncontrolled diabetes mellitus
   1. Non–insulin-dependent diabetes mellitus for the past 8 years
   2. Not currently taking any medication for diabetes
   3. Complains of extreme thirst
   4. Skin parched; lips dry
   5. Random blood sugar 648 mg/dl
   6. Eats one meal a day at local homeless shelter
   7. Blood pressure 94/64 mm Hg; pulse rate 112 beats/min; respirations 12 breaths/min
   8. Polyuria
   9. No ketones on dipstick urinalysis
   10. Lethargic and hypoactive
b. Homeless
   1. Outside temperature 22° F
   2. Body temperature 97.1° F
   3. Wearing jeans and a sweatshirt
   4. Has been sleeping under viaduct
   5. Eats one meal a day at the shelter
c. Draining lesion on foot
   1. Draining lesion 5 by 7 cm on malleolus of right foot
   2. Body temperature 97.1° F
d. Appears defeated
   1. Reluctant to discuss lifestyle and health habits
   2. Poorly groomed with strong body odor
   3. Very passive in interactions with shelter personnel

4. Will not attempt physical responses to examination requests
5. Avoids eye contact with nurse
6. Sits with shoulders slumped, hands hanging at sides
7. States "I'm a loner"
8. States, "God gave up on me a long time ago"
9. Repeatedly apologizes that time and resources are going to a "bum"

At this point it would be a good idea to do a quick review of all the available assessment data. Are any cues that are possibly important in your planning for this client not currently being considered? Because you eliminated some of the general problem areas before you reclustered the data, it is important to quickly review all the cues. This would ensure that no critical cues has been excluded simply because the general problem area in which it would have been clustered has been deleted.

For example, you may have identified abdominal pain as a problem earlier in the critical thinking process, but it is not linked to one of the general problems being considered. This is an example of the need to reexamine your data to be certain that no important cue has been omitted prematurely from consideration. Pain should be investigated, since it may herald a serious impending problem. The client's lack of cooperation and apathy make further investigation of this symptom difficult. The general problem of abdominal pain should be added to the list of problems for immediate consideration.

Many of the cues were eliminated from consideration early in the process. The urgency of Mr. Martin's health status merited an acceleration of the critical thinking process. This accelerated thinking is easier for the experienced nurse than for the novice nurse. The experienced nurse is better able to recognize what can wait and what cannot wait.

4. Before formulating her nursing diagnoses, the student nurse decides to call her clinical instructor to discuss the puzzling signs related to the status of the client's diabetes. Her initial impression was that Mr. Martin was in diabetic ketoacidosis. However, the lack of ketosis substantiated by the negative result of the urine dipstick has her puzzled. Also, diabetic ketoacidosis usually occurs in insulin-dependent diabetics. The client is not on an insulin regimen.

After a brief discussion of the situation, the student and the faculty member conclude that Mr. Martin probably has hyperglycemic hyperosmolar nonketosis (HHNK) rather than diabetic ketoacidosis. The high

mortality rate associated with HHNK makes it imperative that the student arrange transfer for the client to the local hospital as quickly as possible so that a definitive diagnosis can be made.

In this case the nurse must recognize the seriousness of the physiologic cues. It is not critically important that the student pick up the subtle differences between HHNK and ketoacidosis. The nurse is not responsible for the medical diagnosis for Mr. Martin. What is important is that she recognizes the seriousness of his health status and acts swiftly to intervene.

While the student is waiting for the ambulance to arrive to transport Mr. Martin to the hospital, she finishes the nursing diagnostic statements.

The nursing diagnoses for this client include the following:

  a. *Potential complication: Hyperglycemic hyperosmolar nonketosis*
  b. *Hypothermia related to inadequate clothing and prolonged exposure to cold outside temperature as manifested by body temperature of 97.1° F*
  c. *Potential complication: foot lesion*
  d. *Hopelessness related to complex social and health problems as manifested by passivity, failure to respond, lack of eye contact, and dejected posture*
  e. *Pain related to unknown etiology as manifested by grimacing when abdomen palpated*

The diagnosis of *pain* cannot be discarded because the cause of the problem is not known at this time. Further assessment will clarify the cause of the problem.

5. On consideration of the definitions and defining characteristics of the nursing diagnoses under consideration and the collaborative problem statements, you note that all of them are accurate. However, you recognize that the potential complication of HHNK is of highest priority at this time. All other diagnoses are less accurate because they are of a lesser priority.[4]

At this point there is nothing that the nursing student can do related to the client's diabetic complication. However, early in the encounter with Mr. Martin she could have provided him with a blanket to begin the rewarming process. While waiting for the ambulance, the student could put a sterile dressing over the draining foot lesion to prevent further trauma and contamination during transport. She could also try to prepare the client for the impending emergency department experience and the high probability of hospital admission. It would be kind of her to assure him that the health professionals who will be caring for him are genuinely concerned about his welfare and do not sit in judgment of his lifestyle.

6. The case could present a difficult moral dilemma for the nursing student. She admits to herself that she finds the client offensive. She may even believe that he has only himself to blame for his present predicament. However, it is her professional responsibility to set aside her biases and prejudices and provide this very sick man with the best care she has to offer. The student appears to have acted responsibly and humanely. It might be advisable for her to discuss her feelings toward this client with her instructor or a trusted confidante to clarify any lingering issues.

Case Study Twenty-Six

PART TWO

1. The general problem areas for this client at discharge are as follows:

   a. Concern over ability to self-manage diabetes
   b. Underweight
   c. Poor self-image
   d. No supportive family or friends
   e. Poor coping styles
   f. Spiritual distress

2. Data for the identified problem areas would be reclustered as follows:

   a. Concern about ability to self-manage diabetes
     1. Expressed concern over his ability to maintain his prescribed treatment plan
   b. Underweight
     1. Height 5´11˝; weight 154 pounds
   c. Poor self-image
     1. Makes many denigrating remarks about himself and homeless state
   d. No supportive family or friends
     1. Had no visitors during his hospitalization
     2. Made no phone calls
   e. Poor coping styles
     1. Unwilling to discuss his life or the events leading to his homelessness
     2. Coping styles appear to be denial and avoidance
   f. No spiritual beliefs
     1. Refused to see hospital chaplain
     2. States that "God gave up on me a long time ago"

3. Ms. Demarest believed that Mr. Martin was concerned about his ability to manage a fairly sophisticated treatment plan, which made *ineffective management of therapeutic regimen* a valid hypothesis. You believed that this diagnosis was premature and that Mr. Martin should be given the opportunity to manage his treatment plan even though he had some concerns about his ability to do so. You did admit, however, that his circumstances were less than ideal for maintaining tight diabetes control. You and Ms. Demarest compromised by changing the diagnosis to *risk for ineffective management of therapeutic regimen*. This diagnosis would alert the next nurse to watch for this problem and to institute measures to prevent it from becoming a diagnosis.

Because Mr. Martin was extremely dehydrated on admission as a result of the loss of fluid caused by HHNK, he looked extremely drawn and thin. Based on his physical appearance, Ms. Demarest suggested the diagnosis of *altered nutrition: Less than body requirements*. Rehydration and good food during his 10-day hospital stay resulted in his gaining 9 pounds. You consulted a height and weight chart and showed that Mr. Martin, although appearing to be undernourished, actually was in the low range of normal for weight and height. Therefore he did not meet the defining characteristics for this diagnosis, and *altered nutrition: Less than body requirements* was not an accurate diagnosis. Undernourished appearance would not be an appropriate etiology under any circumstance, since it is not a cause of the problem but a sign of it.

You did think that Mr. Martin was a candidate for the diagnosis of *risk for altered nutrition: Less than body requirements* based on his lifestyle, lack of physical and financial access to food, increased nutritional requirements because of a draining foot lesion, and anorexia. Use of this diagnosis would alert other health-care providers to the need for planning of interventions to prevent this risk diagnosis from becoming a diagnosis.

You and Ms. Demarest agreed on the diagnosis of *self-esteem disturbance*. It is an accurate diagnosis based on his self-denigrating statements and comments about worthlessness. You are all hopeful that his improved physical condition, more stable living environment, and job retraining will help improve his self-esteem.

You are puzzled by Ms. Demarest's declaration that *altered family process* is an accurate diagnosis for Mr. Martin. When you ask her for her thinking about this diagnosis, she states that obviously there are problems within the family unit or some family members would have been to the hospital to visit him. When asked if she validated this diagnosis with the client, Ms. Demarest said she did not want to bring it up and make him upset that his family deserted him when he needed them. You suggest that this diagnosis is not accurate because it was not validated by the client or supported by the available data. It is not even known whether Mr. Martin has a family! Reluctantly, Ms. Demarest erases *altered family process* from the chalkboard.

You and Ms. Demarest again agree on the diagnosis of *ineffective individual coping*. In all your dealing with Mr. Martin, at no time did you see him use any positive coping styles. Rather, he used denial and avoidance when confronted with a conflict or decision. At this time, you are not certain of the etiology of the problem. Perhaps Mr. Martin is unaware of any other ways to deal with his problems. Or, perhaps he has no insight into the negative coping styles he is using. Further assessment could identify the etiology of the problem and give direction for future interventions. You feel that this diagnosis is an important one for the community nurse to follow up.

You really have to think about the last hypothesized nursing diagnosis of *spiritual distress*. After reviewing the definition and defining characteristics, you decide that you do not have enough data to make this a diagnosis. You do think that there is enough information suggestive of this diagnosis to warrant keeping it as a possible diagnosis. This way, the diagnosis of *possible spiritual distress* alerts the nurse to gather additional information to either confirm or refute the diagnosis. If the diagnosis were supported by additional data, then appropriate nursing interventions would need to be planned.

4. Ms. Demarest made the following errors in her critical thinking about this client and the nursing diagnoses that she considered accurate:

a. She jumped to the conclusion that Mr. Martin would not be able to manage his treatment plan, despite extensive teaching during his hospitalization. It is always a temptation to predict an outcome based on preconceptions and biases. In this case there was no evidence to support the diagnosis of ineffective management of therapeutic regimen, although it is certainly an area that needs careful monitoring.

b. Physical appearance of a client should not be the only criterion for assigning a diagnosis. In the case of *altered nutrition: Less than body requirements*, the height and weight chart provided the scientific knowledge base to determine that Mr. Martin was not below his ideal body weight, so the diagnosis was not appropriate.

c. Ms. Demarest, being a mother and a daughter, was incensed that none of Mr. Martin's family came to visit him. She again made assumptions that (1) he had a family, (2) they lived in the area, and (3) it bothered Mr. Martin that they did not visit. The diagnosis of *altered family process* requires that there be a change from functional to dysfunctional family process. There

is simply too much missing information to consider the diagnosis. Ms. Demarest failed to validate the diagnosis with the client, which might have shed light on the accuracy of the hypothesized diagnosis.

d. Her final diagnostic error was in projecting her own set of spiritual values on her client. Ms. Demarest is a religious woman who assumes that all people need a higher power in their lives. Mr. Martin's refusal to see the hospital chaplain convinced Ms. Demarest that Mr. Martin was in spiritual distress. His comment about "God giving up on him" is suggestive of a possible problem but not an accurate enough cue to warrant the diagnosis.

Ms. Demarest is an example of a well-meaning, competent nurse who often uses her intuition and personal beliefs to analyze client problems. Had she taken the time to study the definitions and defining characteristics of the various diagnoses she proposed, she would have been more accurate from the beginning. Careful use of the critical thinking process can prevent such diagnostic errors.

5. The nursing diagnoses that would be included on the discharge summary are as follows:

a. *Risk for ineffective management of therapeutic regimen related to complex treatment regimen and limited resources*

b. *Self-esteem disturbance related to homeless state as manifested by self-denigrating comments*

c. *Ineffective individual coping related to unknown etiology as manifested by use of denial and avoidance*

d. *Possible spiritual distress related to homeless state*

e. *Risk for altered nutrition: Less than body requirements related to lack of physical and financial access to food, increased nutritional requirements secondary to anorexia and a draining foot lesion*

6. The diagnosis with the highest priority is *risk for ineffective management of therapeutic regimen*. At this time Mr. Martin's physiologic status is stable and his diabetes in good control. Although the other diagnoses are certainly important, unless he continues to maintain his present stable health state, there would be little progress in these other areas. Once the community health nurse is certain that Mr. Martin can manage his regimen, she can then proceed to plan interventions appropriate to the other diagnoses.

Case Study Twenty-Seven

PART ONE

1. This is a complex client situation for several reasons. First, the client has had a very disabling injury at a time in her life when she should have been active with her peer group. One of the primary developmental tasks at 16 years of age is that of identity versus role confusion. Self-concept is achieved, and peer group plays an important role. The adolescent at this age is preoccupied with the way she appears in the eyes of others as compared with her own self-concept. Erikson describes the psychosocial stages of intimacy versus isolation for the ages 16 to 22 years. Important tasks in this stage include developing an intimate love relationship with another and intimate interpersonal relationships with friends. Without intimacy the individual feels isolated and alone. The nurse applies information from theory of growth and development when assessing the client and planning nursing interventions.

Second, this is a complex case because, although Eileen lives in an environment where there are many people, she makes it clear that she wants to be left alone. Eileen has tried to prevent socialization by placing a sign on her door telling everyone not to bother her. The nurse should explore the reasons for the sign. This exploration may provide additional data to validate an actual nursing diagnosis.

Third, a stage IV pressure ulcer is the most severe degree of ulceration. In this type of pressure ulcer deep tissue destruction extends through the subcutaneous tissue to fascia and possibly involves muscle layers, joint, and bone. There may be necrotic tissue, sinus tract formation, and infection. The complexity of Eileen's stage IV pressure ulcer is increased because of its location and the compounding factors of bowel incontinence, decreased mobility, and questionable nutrition. This degree of pressure ulcer development is significant because of the attendant risk of sepsis.

2. The general problem areas you can identify based on the preceding data are as follows:

    a. Decreased mobility
    b. Pressure ulcer
    c. Lack of age-appropriate social interaction
    d. Bowel incontinence

3. Data are reclustered according to each general problem area as follows:

    a. Decreased mobility
      1. Paraplegic for 6 years
      2. Works as a bookkeeper
      3. Stage IV sacral pressure ulcer
      4. Uses a wheelchair
    b. Pressure ulcer
      1. Stage IV sacral pressure ulcer
      2. Incontinent of very large, loose, unformed stool
      3. Paraplegic
      4. Bookkeeper job requires long periods of sitting
      5. Empty can of Coke and box of cookies at bedside
    c. Lack of age-appropriate social interaction
      1. 22 years old
      2. Lives alone
      3. Bedroom dark (during the middle of the day), curtains drawn, clutter all over the room
      4. Disheveled, unkempt
      5. Has no friends
      6. Has sign on door stating "Do not bother me!"
      7. Mother lives in town but visits rarely
      8. Works as a bookkeeper
    d. Bowel incontinence
      1. Incontinent of very large, loose, unformed stool
      2. Usually manages bowel continence with diet modification and bowel evacuation schedule

4. There are sufficient cues in each of the problem areas to make diagnostic hypotheses; however, there are not enough cues to identify the etiology of each diagnosis. Additional questioning will add to the depth of information required by the nurse to plan individualized interventions. You may ask a different set of questions to obtain additional data. However, for the sake of the case study you should use the following new data:

    a. Decreased mobility
      She has been paraplegic for 6 years. During this time she has held a job and lived independently. You are curious about what is happening

now that makes her decreased mobility a problem—or is it the problem? The following questions come to mind:

1. What is her understanding about the length of time she should remain in one position?

    She has knowledge about changing position regularly but expresses anger and hostility toward mother, co-workers, and health-care providers by refusing to change her sitting position frequently as they each remind her to do so.

2. How does she feel about being paraplegic?

    One could anticipate that she may have unresolved feelings about her disability. Has she ever received counseling to help her deal with her altered mobility or with her feelings surrounding her altered mobility? Is there anyone who serves as a support person to Eileen?

    She expresses hopelessness about her future, says she feels even more immobile than her paraplegia makes her, and does not know what to do about her life.

b. Pressure ulcer

  The following questions may be asked:

1. Is this the first pressure ulcer she has had?

    She has had stage II pressure ulcers before, which resolved with more careful attention to positioning. She has never had a stage IV pressure ulcer before.

2. What has been her self-care routine for preventing pressure ulcers? What does she know about the prevention of pressure ulcers? How long does she sit at work? How long does she stay in bed? Is she changing her position at least every 2 hours?

    She is well aware of the specific care required to prevent pressure ulcers. She usually bathes daily and at that time checks her "tailbone" and heels for signs of redness. She uses a special device in her wheelchair to relieve pressure. She does not have a special mattress. She gets very angry when the nurse asks these questions, indicating that "of course I know what to do but what difference does it make? My life isn't worth anything anyway like this."

3. How has this ulcer been treated? What is the progress? How does she feel about it?

    This ulcer has had a prolonged recovery; surgery, numerous dressing techniques, and instruction about avoiding pressure have been prominent interventions. Eileen has been dealing with this pressure ulcer for at least 4 months, so she feels that her situation is "pretty hopeless."

4. Has she increased her intake of calories and protein to meet the increased needs caused by the severe pressure ulcer?

    She admits to eating "poorly." She verbalizes an understanding about the need for high-calorie, high-protein food intake but does not follow that because "I don't feel like it."

c. Lack of age-appropriate social interaction

    To diagnose this problem, you need to identify that there has been a change in behavior. If she has always had few friends, you would not conclude that a dysfunction is present. Also, if she does not perceive that there is any problem with the absence of friends, you would be remiss in diagnosing a problem. The following questions may be asked:

1. What has her past behavior been with regard to friends?

2. What are her feelings about having friends?

    She has one person who picks her up sometimes for church, but she says she lost all her "so-called friends" after the accident. She speaks with a very angry, sharp voice. She states that she would prefer that people leave her alone rather than feel sorry for her. She adds that she is usually tired anyway after work and likes to sleep when she is home.

d. Bowel incontinence

    When did the loose stools begin? Is this a new development? Does she have any idea what may be causing the loose stools?

    She states that she is "tired of following my routine." She has had only the "diarrhea" today. She thinks it may be due to something she ate yesterday. She has a low-grade fever with a temperature of 100.5° F. The nurse wonders whether Eileen could have a virus or an infection of the pressure ulcer.

Refer to p. 134 for the questions for Part Two.

Case Study Twenty-Seven

PART TWO

1. With the new data, it is possible to identify the following diagnostic hypotheses:

   a. *Impaired physical mobility*
   b. *Impaired skin integrity* or *potential complication: stage IV pressure ulcer*
   c. *Ineffective management of therapeutic regimen*
   d. *Impaired adjustment*
   e. *Hopelessness*
   f. *Ineffective individual coping*
   g. *Impaired home maintenance management*
   h. *Bowel incontinence*

2. You may have selected *impaired physical mobility* as the primary nursing diagnosis because of her paraplegia and obvious limitations in mobility. *Impaired physical mobility* is "a state in which the individual experiences a limitation of ability for independent physical movement."[3] Just looking at the definition you can see that Eileen certainly has impaired mobility; however, when the defining characteristics are examined, the diagnosis does not fit. Eileen is rehabilitated to her maximal functional potential (that is, she is working and living alone). She also does not demonstrate the defining characteristic of inability to purposefully move within the physical environment because she takes care of herself, uses a wheelchair, and maintains a job. Nor does she exhibit a limited range of motion, since she has been performing her activities of daily living.

As you look at all the possible nursing diagnoses and attempt to pinpoint the diagnosis that is of highest priority and is most useful in guiding nursing interventions, keep in mind that her paraplegia is a fact. The nurse can do nothing about it. The nurse must, however, consider whether this factor could be the root problem in Eileen's changed behavior with regard to her self-care. From the data it appears that she had been taking care of herself satisfactorily. Now she is refusing to comply with the nursing and medical treatment plans; she has allowed a serious pressure ulcer to develop; she appears unable or unwilling to do things that would facilitate healing of this pressure ulcer. Therefore one can conclude that impaired physical mobility is best used as an etiology of her problems rather than as a nursing diagnosis.

The nurse has made this home visit to change a dressing on a stage IV sacral pressure ulcer. This degree of pressure ulcer may be diagnosed as *impaired skin integrity* according to the present NANDA definition. Carpenito[5] suggests that a stage IV pressure ulcer may more correctly be labeled a collaborative problem, that is, *potential complication: Stage IV pressure ulcer,* since the nurse would not be able to treat the pressure ulcer independently. The authors recommend the use of *potential complication* in this instance.

In this case the nurse must explore the issues related to the etiology of the pressure ulcer. The data suggest that the client may be applying too much pressure to the ischial area. She works as a bookkeeper (Does she sit for long periods of time?) She also spends a lot of time lying supine in bed (How often does she change position? Does she relieve pressure from the ischial area with the pillows?) The pressure ulcer is clearly related, in part, to her impaired physical mobility, but it may also be related to other factors, including moisture and contamination from bowel incontinence, inadequate nutrition, and psychological and emotional factors.

By looking at the data—both within clusters and across clusters—you cannot help but be struck by the emotional state of this client. It seems that she is not taking care of herself well at all. Several diagnostic hypotheses related to her psychological responses are examined:

   a. *Impaired adjustment*
   b. *Hopelessness*
   c. *Ineffective individual coping*
   d. *Ineffective management of therapeutic regimen*

Impaired adjustment is defined as "the state in which the individual is unable to modify his/her lifestyle/behavior in a manner consistent with a change in health status."[3] The relevant major defining characteristic evidenced by Eileen is her unsuccessful ability to be involved in problem solving or goal setting. Using Lunney's[4] scale of accuracy, this would not be a highly accurate nursing diagnosis, since only one supporting cue is present. *Impaired adjustment* may be an etiology of another problem. It should not be disregarded in your planning.

Another nursing diagnosis to review is *hopelessness,* which is defined as "a subjective state in which an individual sees limited or no alternatives or personal choices available and is unable to mobilize energy on own behalf."[3] The major defining characteristics Eileen displays include passivity and verbal cues such as stating that she feels hopeless and does not know what to do about her life. There are also minor defining characteristics, such as lack of initiative, increased sleep, and lack of involvement in her care. This is a highly accurate diagnosis based on the presence of many relevant cues. Her hopelessness may also be a significant etiology for other nursing diagnoses.

A third nursing diagnosis suggested by the data is *ineffective individual coping*, which is defined by NANDA as "impairment of adaptive behaviors and problem-solving abilities of a person in meeting life's demands and roles."[3] The major defining characteristics in this case are inability to problem-solve and destructive behavior toward self. Also, Eileen's statement that her "life is not worth living like this" is a verbalization of being unable to cope (major defining characteristic). This is an accurate nursing diagnosis.

A fourth nursing diagnosis that is hypothesized based on the cues is *ineffective management of therapeutic regimen*. This is defined by NANDA as "a pattern in which the individual experiences or is at high risk to experience difficulty integrating into daily living a program for treatment of illness and the sequelae of illness that meets specific health goals."[3] One major defining characteristic is present: inappropriate choice of daily living for meeting the goals of a treatment or prevention program. Several minor defining characteristics are present: Acceleration of illness symptoms (that is, pressure ulcer), verbalization that she did not take action to include treatment regimens in daily routines, and verbalization that she did not take action to reduce risk factors for progression of illness and sequelae. Consequently this is also an accurate nursing diagnosis for Eileen.

Impaired home maintenance management is "the inability to independently maintain a safe growth-promoting immediate environment."[3] Although there are no subjective data, there are objective data, such as disorderly surroundings, unwashed cooking equipment and linen, and accumulation of food wastes and bodily wastes, to confirm this diagnosis. The etiology of this diagnosis may be related to Eileen's *hopelessness*.

Bowel incontinence is another diagnosis to be considered in this case. The NANDA definition of *bowel incontinence* is "a state in which an individual experiences a change in normal bowel habits characterized by involuntary passage of stool."[3] The only defining characteristic for *bowel incontinence* is involuntary passage of stool. Eileen indicates that she has managed her bowel continence with diet modification and scheduled bowel evacuation in the past. At this time, however, she is passing large amounts of loose, unformed stool incontinently. Since the defining charac-

teristic is present to support this diagnosis, it is a highly accurate diagnosis. The etiology of this diagnosis seems to be related to discontinuation of her usual bowel regimen. The presence of a low-grade fever must be investigated to determine whether it is related to the diarrhea or whether some other process is ongoing. The nurse also must obtain additional data about Eileen's food intake yesterday, to validate whether this could be the cause of the incontinence.

In writing the priority diagnoses as complete nursing diagnoses, you have several possibilities. The following are identified and the rationales are discussed:

a. *Potential complication: Stage IV pressure ulcer*
   No related factors need to be stated when writing a collaborative problem.[5]

   If you chose to use the NANDA-approved diagnosis, you would write it as follows: *Impaired skin integrity related to prolonged pressure, moisture, and inadequate nutrition as manifested by stage IV pressure ulcer.*

b. *Ineffective management of therapeutic regimen related to impaired physical mobility, impaired adjustment, and hopelessness as manifested by development of stage IV pressure ulcer and reluctance to participate in treatment plan*

After your thorough analysis of the data, you conclude that one of the client's primary problems is that she is not taking care of herself; she is not following the treatment plan. The complex etiology of this diagnosis must be addressed to effectively treat this nursing diagnosis.

You may have chosen to identify four separate nursing diagnoses here (*ineffective management of therapeutic regimen; impaired physical mobility; impaired adjustment;* and *hopelessness*), instead of using one nursing diagnosis with several other diagnoses used as etiologies. That is not incorrect, and that is often what a novice diagnostician might do because beginners see things as discreet items.

With increased knowledge and skill in nursing and in making nursing diagnoses, you may identify the interrelationships between diagnostic labels more easily and feel comfortable in writing this type of diagnostic statement. Gordon[2] stresses that when you use a diagnostic label as an etiology you must be just as rigorous in the choice of that label. To say that one diagnostic label is the problem and another diagnostic label is the etiology requires application of theory, research findings, experience, or a combination of these. The diagnostic term (label) is useful as an etiology because this name is clear and concise and a sufficient cluster of signs and symptoms can be documented to justify its presence.

c. *Ineffective individual coping related to hopelessness and complex medical problems as manifested by verbalization of despair*

Eileen's statement of life not being worth anything now is a highly relevant cue that must be given immediate attention. The nurse's recognition of this cue will result in a plan that includes listening, offering support, assisting with problem solving, and referral to an appropriate mental health professional for treatment beyond the nurse's scope of practice.

d. *Impaired home maintenance management related to hopelessness as manifested by disorderly and unclean living environment*

Nursing interventions would need to be planned to alleviate the hygiene problems created by her hopelessness at this time.

e. *Bowel incontinence related to discontinuation of usual bowel regimen as manifested by large, unformed incontinent stool*

Because of the presence of a stage IV pressure ulcer, Eileen's bowel incontinence takes on greater importance. The nurse will work with Eileen to help her reestablish her previously effective bowel regimen.

3. It is important to consider the context in which this nursing care takes place. The nurse is seeing Eileen in her home. This may affect the dynamics of the therapeutic relationship. Eileen is "on her own turf." The nurse recalls information about how to maintain therapeutic communication and establish therapeutic relationships. This is basic information in nursing; however, the skills involved in therapeutic communication and in establishing therapeutic relationships are developed over time in a variety of situations.

The darkness of Eileen's bedroom is both a contextual cue and a factor to be considered when examining and caring for the client. What does the cue suggest to you? It may suggest that the client is depressed and that she is trying to shut herself off from the environment. The cue must be validated with Eileen. In addition, the nurse needs good lighting to provide the best care. However, the nurse should ask Eileen about the light: "Does it bother you?" "May I turn it on while I do your dressing change?"—and so forth.

Home nursing is different from hospital nursing in many ways, but one significant way is in the independent practice of the nurse. The nurse has no other professional immediately available for assistance or consultation. If there are questions or if assistance is needed, the nurse needs to telephone someone.

In the home setting the nurse provides nursing care and then leaves. This makes it difficult to follow up with immediate evaluation or observations. It may be necessary to establish ongoing telephone follow-up with the client to gain information about the effectiveness of nursing intervention or the client's changing needs.

AUTHORS' POSTSCRIPT: CONSEQUENCES OF FAILURE TO MAKE CORRECT DIAGNOSES

This case was based on a real-life situation. The nurses caring for Eileen worked for a home nursing agency. The nurses were involved in treating the pressure ulcer. No additional data were collected; thus neither nursing diagnoses nor etiologic factors were ever identified. Therefore there was no nursing intervention to treat what we can see from this case study analysis were the major nursing diagnoses for this client: *Ineffective management of therapeutic regimen related to impaired physical mobility, impaired adjustment, hopelessness* and *ineffective individual coping related to hopelessness and complex medical problems as manifested by verbalization of despair.*

An important question to consider when you are providing nursing care is the following: "What would be the consequences if I do not make the correct nursing diagnosis?" The answer is as follows: If accurate nursing diagnoses are not made, the rest of the nursing process will not be completed; therefore the appropriate nursing care is not delivered.

In the case of Eileen the client continued to have contamination of her pressure ulcer, continued to eat poorly, and continued to be uninvolved in her care. Sepsis soon resulted from infection of the pressure ulcer, and she proceeded to go into septic shock in the hospital. She died a short time later.

In reviewing this tragic outcome, it is important to ask: "What went wrong?" The glaring answer is that the diagnostic reasoning process was not used with this client. As a result, an unsatisfactory level of nursing was practiced. The final result was that the client was denied effective nursing care.

This case serves as an example of the ultimate outcome of failure to use a rigorous diagnostic reasoning process. The authors hope this workbook will help develop better diagnostic skills in all nurses: *Nursing diagnosis is the pivotal focus for the whole process of nursing.*

Appendixes

Selected NANDA-Approved Nursing Diagnoses, Definitions, and Defining Characteristics

Activity Intolerance

Definition

A state in which an individual has insufficient physiological or psychological energy to endure to complete required or desired daily activities.

Defining Characteristics

Verbal report of fatigue or weakness*, abnormal heart rate or blood pressure response to activity, exertional discomfort or dyspnea, electrocardiographic changes reflecting arrhythmias or ischemia.

---

*Critical

Adjustment, Impaired

Definition

The state in which the individual is unable to modify his/her lifestyle/behavior in a manner consistent with a change in health status.

Defining Characteristics

Major: Verbalization of nonacceptance of health status change; nonexistent or unsuccessful ability to be involved in problem solving or goal setting.

Minor: Lack of movement toward independence; extended period of shock, disbelief, or anger regarding health status change; lack of future-oriented thinking.

Airway Clearance, Ineffective

Definition

A state in which an individual is unable to clear secretions or obstructions from the respiratory tract to maintain airway patency.

Defining Characteristics

Abnormal breath sounds (rales [crackles], rhonchi [wheezes]); changes in rate or depth of respiration; tachypnea; cough, effective/ineffective, with or without sputum; cyanosis; dyspnea.

Anxiety

Definition

A vague, uneasy feeling whose source is often nonspecific or unknown to the individual.

Defining Characteristics

Subjective: Increased tension; apprehension; painful and persistent increased helplessness; uncertainty; fearful; scared; regretful; overexcited; rattled; distressed; jittery; feelings of inadequacy; shakiness; fear of unspecific consequences; expressed concerns due to change in life events; worried; anxious.

Objective: Sympathetic stimulation-cardiovascular excitation,* superficial vasoconstriction, pupil dilation; restlessness; insomnia; glancing about; poor eye contact; trembling/hand tremors; extraneous movement (foot shuffling; hand/arm movements); facial tension; voice quivering; focus on self; increased wariness; increased perspiration.

---

*Critical

Aspiration, Risk for
Definition
The state in which an individual is at risk for entry of gastrointestinal secretions, oropharyngeal secretions, or solids or fluids into tracheobronchial passages.

Defining Characteristics
Presence of risk factors such as: Reduced level of consciousness; depressed cough and gag reflexes; presence of tracheostomy or endotracheal tube; incomplete lower esophageal sphincter; gastrointestinal tubes; tube feedings; medication administration; situations hindering elevation of upper body; increased intragastric pressure; increased gastric residual; decreased gastrointestinal motility; delayed gastric emptying; impaired swallowing; facial/oral/neck surgery or trauma; wired jaws.

Body Image Disturbance
Definition
Disruption in the way one perceives one's body image.

Defining Characteristics
A or B must be present to justify the diagnosis of Body Image Disturbance. A = Verbal response to actual or perceived change in structure and/or function; B = nonverbal response to actual or perceived change in structure and/or function. The following clinical manifestations may be used to validate the presence of A or B.

Objective: Missing body part; actual change in structure and/or function; not looking at body part; not touching body part; hiding or overexposing body part (intentional or unintentional); trauma to nonfunctioning part; change in social involvement; change in ability to estimate spatial relationship of body to environment.

Subjective: Verbalization of: Change in lifestyle; fear of rejection or of reaction by others; focus on past strength, function, or appearance; negative feelings about body; feelings of helplessness, hopelessness, or powerlessness; preoccupation with change or loss; emphasis on remaining strengths, heightened achievement; extension of body boundary to incorporate environmental objects; personalization of part or loss by name; depersonalization of part or loss by impersonal pronouns; refusal to verify actual change.

Body Temperature, Risk for Altered
Definition
The state in which the individual is at risk for failure to maintain body temperature within normal range.

Defining Characteristics
Presence of risk factors such as: Extremes of age; extremes of weight; exposure to cold/cool or warm/hot environments; dehydration; inactivity or vigorous activity; medications causing vasoconstriction/vasodilation; altered metabolic rate; sedation; inappropriate clothing for environmental temperature; illness or trauma affecting temperature regulation.

Bowel Incontinence
Definition
A state in which an individual experiences a change in normal bowel habits characterized by involuntary passage of stool.

Defining Characteristics
Involuntary passage of stool.

Breastfeeding, Ineffective
Definition
The state in which a mother, infant, or child experiences dissatisfaction or difficulty with the breastfeeding process.

Defining Characteristics
Major: Unsatisfactory breastfeeding process.

Minor: Actual or perceived inadequate milk supply; infant inability to attach onto maternal breast correctly; no observable signs of oxytocin release; observable signs of inadequate milk intake; nonsustained suckling at the breast; insufficient emptying of each breast per feeding; persistence of sore nipples beyond the first week of breastfeeding; insufficient opportunity for suckling at the breast; infant exhibiting fussiness and crying within the first hour after breastfeeding; unresponsive to other comfort measures; infant arching and crying at the breast; resisting latching on.

Breastfeeding, Interrupted
Definition
A break in the continuity of the breastfeeding process as a result of inability or inadvisability to put baby to breast for feeding.

Defining Characteristics
Major: Infant does not receive nourishment at the breast for some or all of feedings.

Minor: Maternal desire to maintain lactation and provide (or eventually provide) her breastmilk for her infant's nutritional needs; separation of mother and infant; lack of knowledge regarding expression and storage of breastmilk.

Breathing Pattern, Ineffective
Definition
The state in which an individual's inhalation and/or exhalation pattern does not enable adequate pulmonary inflation or emptying.

Defining Characteristics
Dyspnea; shortness of breath; tachypnea; fremitus; abnormal arterial blood gas; cyanosis; cough; nasal flaring; respiratory depth changes; assumption of 3-point position; pursed-lip breathing/prolonged expiratory phase; increased anteroposterior chest diameter; use of accessory muscles; altered chest excursion.

Cardiac Output, Decreased
Definition
A state in which the blood pumped by an individual's heart is sufficiently reduced that it is inadequate to meet the needs of the body's tissues.

Defining Characteristics
Variations in blood pressure readings; arrhythmias; fatigue; jugular vein distention; color changes, skin and mucous membranes; oliguria; decreased peripheral pulses; cold, clammy skin; rales; dyspnea, orthopnea; restlessness.

Caregiver Role Strain
Definition
A caregiver's felt difficulty in performing the family caregiver role.

*Defining Characteristics**
Caregivers report they: Do not have enough resources to provide the care needed; find it hard to do specific caregiving activities; worry about such things as the care receiver's health and emotional state, having to put the care receiver in an institution, and about who will care for the care receiver if something should happen to the caregiver; feel that caregiving interferes with other important roles in their lives; feel loss because the care receiver is like a different person compared to before caregiving began or, in the case of a child, that the care receiver was never the child the caregiver expected; feel family conflict around issues of providing care; feel stress or nervousness in their relationship with the care receiver; feel depressed.

---

*80% of caregivers report one or more of defining characteristics.

Caregiver Role Strain, Risk for
Definition
A caregiver is vulnerable for felt difficulty in performing the family caregiver role.

Risk Factors
Pathophysiologic: Illness severity of the care receiver; addiction or codependency; premature birth/congenital defect; discharge of family member with significant home care needs; caregiver health impairment; unpredictable illness course or instability in the care receiver's health; caregiver is female; psychological or cognitive problems in care receiver.

Developmental: Caregiver is not developmentally ready for caregiver role, e.g., a young adult needing to provide care for middle-aged parent; developmental delay or retardation of the care receiver or caregiver.

Psychological: Marginal family adaptation or dysfunction prior to the caregiving situation; marginal caregiver's coping patterns; past history of poor relationship between caregiver and care receiver; caregiver is spouse; care receiver exhibits deviant, bizarre behavior.

Situational: Presence of abuse or violence; presence of situational stressors that normally affect families, such as significant loss, disaster or crisis, poverty or economic vulnerability, major life events, e.g., birth, hospitalization, leaving home, returning home, marriage, divorce, employment, retirement, death; duration of caregiving required; inadequate physical environment for providing care, e.g., housing, transportation, community services, equipment; family/caregiver isolation; lack of respite and recreation for caregiver; inexperience with caregiving; caregiver's competing role commitments; complexity/amount of caregiving responsibility.

Confusion, Acute
Definition
The abrupt onset of a cluster of global, transient changes and disturbances in attention, cognition, psychomotor activity level of consciousness, and/or sleep/wake cycle.

Defining Characteristics
Major: Fluctuation in cognition; fluctuation in sleep/wake cycle; fluctuation in level of consciousness; fluctuation in psychomotor activity; increased agitation

or restlessness; misperceptions; lack of motivation to initiate and/or follow through with goal-directed or purposeful behavior.

Minor: Hallucinations.

Confusion, Chronic
Definition
An irreversible, long-standing and/or progressive deterioration of intellect and personality characterized by decreased ability to interpret environmental stimuli, decreased capacity for intellectual thought processes and manifested by disturbances of memory, orientation, and behavior.

Defining Characteristics
Major: Clinical evidence of organic impairment; altered interpretation/response to stimuli; progressive/long-standing cognitive impairment.

Minor: No change in level of consciousness; impaired socialization; impaired memory (short term, long term); altered personality.

Constipation
Definition
A state in which an individual experiences a change in normal bowel habits characterized by a decrease in frequency and/or passage of hard, dry stools.

Defining Characteristics
Decreased activity level; frequency less than usual pattern; hard formed stools; palpable mass; reported feeling of pressure in rectum; reported feeling of rectal fullness; straining at stool.

Constipation, Perceived
Definition
The state in which an individual makes a self-diagnosis of constipation and ensures a daily bowel movement through abuse of laxatives, enemas, and suppositories.

Defining Characteristics
Major: Expectation of a daily bowel movement with the resulting overuse of laxatives, enemas, and suppositories; expected passage of stool at same time every day.

Constipation, Colonic
Definition
The state in which an individual's pattern of elimination is characterized by hard, dry stool that results from a delay in passage of food residue.

Defining Characteristics
Major: Decreased frequency; hard, dry stool; straining at stool; painful defecation; abdominal distention; palpable mass.

Minor: Rectal pressure; headache, appetite impairment; abdominal pain.

Coping, Ineffective Individual
Definition
Impairment of adaptive behaviors and problem-solving abilities of a person in meeting life's demands and roles.

Defining Characteristics
Verbalization of inability to cope or inability to ask for help; inability to meet role expectations; inability to meet basic needs; inability to problem-solve; alteration in societal participation; destructive behavior toward self or others; inappropriate use of defense mechanisms; change in usual communication patterns; verbal manipulation; high illness rate; high rate of accidents.

---

*Critical

Coping, Defensive
Definition
The state in which an individual repeatedly projects falsely positive self-evaluation based on a self-protective pattern that defends against underlying perceived threats to positive self-regard.

Defining Characteristics
Major: Denial of obvious problems/weaknesses; projection of blame/responsibility; rationalizes failures; hypersensitive to slight/criticism; grandiosity.

Minor: Superior attitude toward others; difficulty establishing/maintaining relationships; hostile laughter or ridicule of others; difficulty in reality-testing perceptions; lack of follow-through or participation in treatment or therapy.

Coping, Ineffective Family: Disabling
Definition
Behavior of significant person (family member or other primary person) that disables his or her own capacities and the capacity to effectively address tasks essential to either person's adaptation to the health challenge.

Defining Characteristics
Neglectful care of the client in regard to basic human needs and/or illness treatment; distortion of reality regarding the health problem, including extreme de-

nial about its existence or severity; intolerance; rejection; abandonment; desertion; carrying on usual routines, disregarding needs; psychosomaticism; taking on illness signs of client; decisions and actions by family that are detrimental to economic or social well-being; agitation, depression, aggression, hostility; impaired restructuring of a meaningful life for self, impaired individualization, prolonged overconcern for client; neglectful relationships with other family members; client's development of helpless, inactive dependence.

Coping, Ineffective Family: Compromised
Definition
A usually supportive primary person (family member or close friend) is providing insufficient, ineffective, or compromised support, comfort, assistance, or encouragement that may be needed by the client to manage or master adaptive tasks related to his or her health challenge.

Defining Characteristics
Subjective: Client expresses or confirms a concern or complaint about significant other's response to his or her health problem; significant person describes preoccupation with personal reaction (e.g., fear, anticipatory grief, guilt, anxiety to illness, disability, or to other situational or developmental crises); significant person describes or confirms an inadequate understanding or knowledge base that interferes with effective assistive or supportive behaviors.

Objective: Significant person attempts assistive or supportive behaviors with less than satisfactory results; significant person withdraws or enters into limited or temporary personal communication with the client at the time of need; significant person displays protective behavior disproportionate (too little or too much) to the abilities or need for autonomy.

Decisional Conflict
Definition
The state of uncertainty about course of action to be taken when choice among competing actions involves risk, loss, or challenge to personal life values.

Defining Characteristics
Major: Verbalized uncertainty about choices; verbalization of undesired consequences of alternative actions being considered; vacillation between alternative choices; delayed decision making.

Minor: Verbalized feeling of distress while attempting a decision; self-focusing; physical signs of distress or tension (increased heart rate, increased muscle tension, restlessness, etc.); questioning personal values and beliefs while attempting a decision.

Denial, Ineffective
Definition
The state of a conscious or unconscious attempt to disavow the knowledge or meaning of an event to reduce anxiety/fear to the detriment of health.

Defining Characteristics
Major: Delays seeking or refuses health care attention to the detriment of health; does not perceive personal relevance of symptoms or danger.

Minor: Uses home remedies (self-treatment) to relieve symptoms; does not admit fear of death or invalidism; minimizes symptoms; displaces source of symptoms to other organs; unable to admit impact of disease on life pattern; makes dismissive gestures or comments when speaking of distressing events; displaces fear of impact of the condition; displays inappropriate affect.

Diarrhea
Definition
A state in which an individual experiences a change in normal bowel habits characterized by the frequent passage of loose, fluid, unformed stools.

Defining Characteristics
Abdominal pain, cramping; increased frequency; increased frequency of bowel sounds; loose, liquid stools; urgency.

Other Possible Characteristics
Change in color.

Disuse Syndrome, Risk for
Definition
A state in which an individual is at risk for deterioration of body systems as the result of prescribed or unavoidable musculoskeletal inactivity.*

Defining Characteristics
Presence of risk factors such as: Paralysis; mechanical immobilization; prescribed immobilization, severe pain; altered level of consciousness.

---

*Complications from immobility can include pressure ulcer; constipation; stasis of pulmonary secretions; thrombosis; urinary tract infection/retention; decreased strength/endurance; orthostatic hypotension; decreased range of joint motion; disorientation; body image disturbance and powerlessness.

Diversional Activity Deficit

Definition

The state in which an individual experiences a decreased stimulation from (or interest or engagement in) recreational or leisure activities.

Defining Characteristics

Patient's statements regarding: Boredom, wish there was something to do, to read, etc.; usual hobbies cannot be undertaken in hospital.

Dysreflexia

Definition

The state in which an individual with a spinal cord injury at T7 or above experiences a life-threatening uninhibited sympathetic response of the nervous system to a noxious stimulus.

Defining Characteristics

Major: Individual with spinal cord injury (T7 or above) with: Paroxysmal hypertension (sudden periodic elevated blood pressure in which systolic pressure is over 140 mm Hg and diastolic is above 90 mm Hg); bradycardia or tachycardia (pulse rate of less than 60 or more than 100 beats per minute); diaphoresis (above the injury); red splotches on skin (above the injury); pallor (below the injury); headache (a diffuse pain in different portions of the head and not confined to any nerve distribution area).

Minor: Chilling; conjunctival congestion; Horner's syndrome (contraction of the pupil, partial ptosis of the eyelid, enophthalmos and sometimes loss of sweating over the affected side of the face); paresthesia; pilomotor reflex (gooseflesh formation when skin is cooled); blurred vision; chest pain; metallic taste in mouth; nasal congestion.

Environmental Interpretation Syndrome, Impaired

Definition

Consistent lack of orientation to person, place, time or circumstances over more than 3 to 6 months, necessitating a protective environment.

Defining Characteristics

Major: Consistent disorientation in known and unknown environments; chronic confusional states.

Minor: Loss of occupation or social functioning from memory decline; inability to follow simple directions, instructions; inability to reason; inability to concentrate; slow in responding to questions.

Family Processes, Altered

Definition

The state in which a family that normally functions effectively experiences a dysfunction.

Defining Characteristics

Family system unable to meet physical needs of its members; family system unable to meet emotional needs of its members; family system unable to meet spiritual needs of its members; parents do not demonstrate respect for each other's views on child-rearing practices; inability to express/accept wide range of feelings; inability to express/accept feelings of members; family unable to meet security needs of its members; inability of the family members to relate to each other for mutual growth and maturation; family uninvolved in community activities; inability to accept/receive help appropriately; rigidity in function and roles; a family not demonstrating respect for individuality and autonomy of its members; family unable to adapt to change/deal with traumatic experience constructively; family failing to accomplish current/past developmental task; unhealthy family decision-making process; failure to send and receive clear messages; inappropriate boundary maintenance; inappropriate/poorly communicated family rules, rituals, symbols; unexamined family myths; inappropriate level and direction of energy.

Family Processes, Altered: Alcoholism

Definition

The state in which the psychosocial, spiritual, and physiologic functions of the family unit are chronically disorganized, leading to conflict, denial of problems, resistance to change, ineffective problem-solving, and a series of self-perpetuating crises.

Defining Characteristics

Major:

Feelings: Decreased self-esteem/worthlessness; anger/suppressed rage; frustration; powerlessness; anxiety/tension/distress; insecurity; repressed emotions; responsibility for alcoholic's behavior; lingering resentment; shame/embarrassment; hurt; unhappiness; guilt; emotional isolation/loneliness; vulnerability; mistrust; hopelessness; rejection.

Roles and relationships: Deterioration in family relationships/disturbed family dynamics; ineffective spousal communication/marital problems; altered role function/disruption of family roles; inconsistent parenting/low perception of parental support; family denial; intimacy dysfunction; chronic family problems; closed communication systems.

Behaviors: Expression of anger inappropriately; difficulty with intimate relationships; loss of control of drinking; impaired communication; ineffective problem-solving skills; enabling to maintain drinking; inability to meet emotional needs of its members; manipulation; dependency; criticizing; alcohol abuse; broken promises; rationalization/denial of problems; refusal to get help/inability to accept and receive help appropriately; blaming; inadequate understanding or knowledge of alcoholism.

Minor:

Feelings: Being different from other people; depression; hostility; fear; emotional control by others; confusion; dissatisfaction; loss; misunderstood; abandonment; confused love and pity; moodiness; failure; being unloved; lack of identity.

Roles and relationships: Triangulating family relationships; reduced ability of family members to relate to each other for mutual growth and maturation; lack of skills necessary for relationships; lack of cohesiveness; disrupted family rituals; family unable to meet security needs of its members; family does not demonstrate respect for individuality and autonomy of its members; pattern of rejection; economic problems; neglected obligations.

Behaviors: Inability to meet spiritual needs of its members; inability to express or accept wide range of feelings; orientation toward tension relief rather than achievement of goals; family special occasions are alcohol centered; escalating conflict; lying; contradictory, paradoxic communication; lack of dealing with conflict; harsh self-judgement; isolation; nicotine addiction; difficulty having fun; self-blaming; unresolved grief; controlling communication/power struggles; inability to adapt to change; immaturity; stress-related physical illnesses; inability to deal with traumatic experiences constructively; seeking approval and affirmation; lack of reliability; disturbances in academic performance in children; disturbances in concentration; chaos; substance abuse other than alcohol; failure to accomplish current or past developmental tasks/difficulty with life-cycle transitions; verbal abuse of spouse or parent; agitation; diminished physical contact.

Fatigue

Definition

An overwhelming sustained sense of exhaustion and decreased capacity for physical and mental work.

Defining Characteristics

Major: Verbalization of an unremitting and overwhelming lack of energy; inability to maintain usual routines.

Minor: Perceived need for additional energy to accomplish routine tasks; increase in physical complaints; emotionally labile or irritable; impaired ability to concentrate; decreased performance; lethargic or listless; disinterest in surroundings/introspection; decreased libido; accident prone.

Fear

Definition

Feeling of dread related to an identifiable source that the person validates.

Defining Characteristics

Ability to identify object of fear.

Fluid Volume Excess

Definition

The state in which an individual experiences increased fluid retention and edema.

Defining Characteristics

Edema; effusion; anasarca; weight gain; shortness of breath, orthopnea; intake greater than output; S_3 heart sound; pulmonary congestion (as seen on chest x-ray); abnormal breath sounds, rales (crackles); change in respiratory pattern; change in mental status; decreased hemoglobin and hematocrit; blood pressure changes; central venous pressure changes; pulmonary artery pressure changes; jugular vein distention; positive hepatojugular reflex; oliguria; urine specific gravity changes; azotemia; altered electrolytes; restlessness and anxiety.

Fluid Volume Deficit

Definition

The state in which an individual experiences vascular, cellular, or intracellular dehydration.

Defining Characteristics

Change in urine output; change in urine concentration; sudden weight loss or gain; decreased venous filling; hemoconcentration; change in serum sodium.

Other Possible Characteristics

Hypotension; thirst; increased pulse rate; decreased skin turgor; decreased pulse volume/pressure; change in mental state; increased body temperature; dry skin; dry mucous membranes; weakness.

Fluid Volume Deficit, Risk for

Definition

The state in which an individual is at risk of experiencing vascular, cellular, or intracellular dehydration.

Defining Characteristics

Presence of risk factors such as: Extremes of age; extremes of weight; excessive losses through normal routes, e.g., diarrhea; loss of fluid through abnormal routes, e.g., indwelling tubes; deviations affecting access to or intake or absorption of fluids, e.g., physical immobility; factors influencing fluid needs, e.g., hypermetabolic state; knowledge deficiency related to fluid volume; medications, e.g., diuretics.

Gas Exchange, Impaired

Definition

The state in which the individual experiences a decreased passage of oxygen and/or carbon dioxide between the alveoli of the lungs and the vascular system.

Defining Characteristics

Confusion; somnolence; restlessness; irritability; inability to move secretions; hypercapnea; hypoxia.

Grieving, Anticipatory

Definition

Intellectual and emotional responses and behaviors by which individuals work through the process of modifying self-concept based on the perception of potential loss.

Defining Characteristics

Potential loss of significant object; expression of distress at potential loss; denial of potential loss; guilt; anger; sorrow, choked feelings; changes in eating habits; alterations in sleep patterns; alterations in activity level; altered libido; altered communication patterns.

Grieving, Dysfunctional

Definition

Extended, unsuccessful use of intellectual and emotional responses by which individuals attempt to work through the process of modifying self-concept based on the perception of loss.

Defining Characteristics

Verbal expression of distress at loss; denial of loss; expression of guilt; expression of unresolved issues; anger; sadness; crying; difficulty in expressing loss; alterations in: eating habits, sleep patterns, dream patterns, activity level, libido; idealization of lost object; reliving of past experiences; interference with life functioning; developmental regression; labile affect; alterations in concentration and/or pursuits of tasks.

Health Maintenance, Altered

Definition

Inability to identify, manage, and/or seek out help to maintain health.

Defining Characteristics

Demonstrated lack of knowledge regarding basic health practices; demonstrated lack of adaptive behaviors to internal/external environmental changes; reported or observed inability to take responsibility for meeting basic health practices in any or all functional pattern areas; history of lack of health-seeking behavior; expressed interest in improving health behaviors; reported or observed lack of equipment, financial and/or other resources; reported or observed impairment of personal support systems.

Health Seeking Behaviors

Definition

A state in which an individual in stable health is actively seeking ways to alter personal health habits and/or the environment in order to move toward a higher level of health.*

Defining Characteristics

Major: Expressed or observed desire to seek a higher level of wellness.

Minor: Expressed or observed desire for increased control of health practice; expression of concern about current environmental conditions on health status; stated or observed unfamiliarity with wellness community resources; demonstrated or observed lack of knowledge in health promotion behaviors.

---

*Stable health status is defined as: Age-appropriate illness prevention measures are achieved, client reports good or excellent health, and signs and symptoms of disease, if present, are controlled.

Home Maintenance Management, Impaired

Definition

Inability to independently maintain a safe growth-promoting immediate environment.

Defining Characteristics

Subjective: Household members express difficulty in maintaining their home in a comfortable fashion*:

household members request assistance with home maintenance*; household members describe outstanding debts or financial crises.*

Objective: Disorderly surroundings; unwashed or unavailable cooking equipment, clothes, or linen*; accumulation of dirt, food wastes, or hygienic wastes; offensive odors*; inappropriate household temperature; overtaxed family members, e.g., exhausted, anxious*; lack of necessary equipment or aids; presence of vermin or rodents; repeated hygienic disorders, infestations, or infections.*

_____
*Critical

Hopelessness
Definition
A subjective state in which an individual sees limited or no alternatives or personal choices available and is unable to mobilize energy on own behalf.

Defining Characteristics
Major: Passivity, decreased verbalization; decreased affect; verbal cues (despondent content, "I can't," sighing).

Minor: Lack of initiative; decreased response to stimuli; decreased affect; turning away from speaker; closing eyes; shrugging in response to speaker; decreased appetite; increased/decreased sleep; lack of involvement in care/passively allowing care.

Hyperthermia
Definition
A state in which an individual's body temperature is elevated above his/her normal range.

Defining Characteristics
Major: Increase in body temperature above normal range.

Minor: Flushed skin; warm to touch; increased respiratory rate; tachycardia; seizures/convulsions.

Hypothermia
Definition
The state in which an individual's body temperature is reduced below normal range.

Defining Characteristics
Major: Reduction in body temperature below normal range; shivering (mild); cool skin; pallor (moderate).

Minor: Slow capillary refill; tachycardia; cyanotic nail beds; hypertension; piloerection.

Incontinence, Stress
Definition
The state in which an individual experiences a loss of urine of less than 50 ml occurring with increased abdominal pressure.

Defining Characteristics
Major: Reported or observed dribbling with increased abdominal pressure.

Minor: Urinary urgency; urinary frequency (more often than every 2 hours).

Incontinence, Reflex
Definition
The state in which an individual experiences an involuntary loss of urine, occurring at somewhat predictable intervals when a specific bladder volume is reached.

Defining Characteristics
Major: No awareness of bladder filling; no urge to void or feelings of bladder fullness; uninhibited bladder contraction/spasm at regular intervals.

Incontinence, Urge
Definition
The state in which an individual experiences involuntary passage of urine occurring soon after a strong sense of urgency to void.

Defining Characteristics
Major: Urinary urgency; frequency (voiding more often than every 2 hours); bladder contracture/spasm.

Minor: Nocturia (more than two times per night); voiding in small amounts (less than 100 ml) or in large amounts (more than 550 ml); inability to reach toilet in time.

Incontinence, Functional
Definition
The state in which an individual experiences an involuntary, unpredictable passage of urine.

Defining Characteristics
Major: Urge to void or bladder contractions sufficiently strong to result in loss of urine before reaching an appropriate receptacle.

Incontinence, Total

Definition
The state in which an individual experiences a continuous and unpredictable loss of urine.

Defining Characteristics
Major: Constant flow of urine occurs at unpredictable times without distention or uninhibited bladder contractions/spasm; unsuccessful incontinence refractory treatments; nocturia.

Minor: Lack of perineal or bladder-filling awareness; unawareness of incontinence.

Infection, Risk for

Definition
The state in which an individual is at increased risk for being invaded by pathogenic organisms.

Defining Characteristics
Presence of risk factors such as: Inadequate primary defenses (broken skin, traumatized tissue, decrease in ciliary action, stasis of body fluids, change in pH secretions, altered peristalsis); inadequate secondary defenses (e.g., decreased hemoglobin, leukopenia, suppressed inflammatory response) and immunosuppression; inadequate acquired immunity; tissue destruction and increased environmental exposure; chronic disease; invasive procedures; malnutrition; pharmaceutical agents; trauma; rupture of amniotic membranes; insufficient knowledge to avoid exposure to pathogens.

Injury, Risk for

Definition
A state in which the individual is at risk of injury as a result of environmental conditions interacting with the individual's adaptive and defensive resources.

Defining Characteristics
Presence of risk factors such as:
Internal: Biochemical, regulatory function (sensory dysfunction; integrative dysfunction; effector dysfunction; tissue hypoxia) malnutrition; immune-auto-immune dysfunction; abnormal blood profile (leukocytosis/leukopenia; altered clotting factors; thrombocytopenia; sickle cell, thalassemia; decreased hemoglobin); physical (broken skin, altered mobility); developmental age (physiologic, psychosocial) psychological (affective, orientation.)

External: Biological (immunization level of community, microorganism); chemical (pollutants, poisons, drugs, pharmaceutical agents, alcohol, caffeine, nicotine, preservatives, cosmetics and dyes), nutrients (vitamins, food types); physical (design, structure, and arrangement of community, building, and/or equipment); mode of transport/transportation; people/provider (nosocomial agents; staffing patterns; cognitive, affective, and psychomotor factors.)

Knowledge Deficit

Definition
Absence or deficiency of cognitive information related to specific topic.

Defining Characteristics
Verbalization of the problem; inaccurate follow-through of instruction; inaccurate performance of test; inappropriate or exaggerated behaviors, e.g., hysterical, hostile, agitated, apathetic.

Loneliness, Risk for

Definition
A subjective state in which an individual is at risk of experiencing vague dysphoria.

Management of Therapeutic Regimen, Ineffective (Individual)

Definition
A pattern of regulating and integrating into daily living a program for treatment of illness and the sequelae of illness that are unsatisfactory for meeting specific health goals.

Defining Characteristics
Major: Choices of daily living ineffective for meeting the goals of a treatment or prevention program.

Minor: Acceleration (expected or unexpected) of illness symptoms; verbalized desire to manage the treatment of illness and prevention of sequelae; verbalized difficulty with regulation/integration of one or more prescribed regimens for treatment of illness and its effects or prevention of complications; verbalized that did not take action to include treatment regimens in daily routines; verbalized that did not take action to reduce risk factors for progression of illness and sequelae.

Management of Therapeutic Regimen: Families, Ineffective

Definition
A pattern of regulating and integrating into family processes a program for treatment of illness and the sequelae of illness that are unsatisfactory for meeting specific health goals.

Defining Characteristics
Major: Inappropriate family activities for meeting the goals of a treatment or prevention program.

Minor: Acceleration (expected or unexpected) of illness symptoms of a family member; lack of attention to illness and its sequelae; verbalized desire to manage the treatment of illness and prevention of the sequelae; verbalized difficulty with regulation/integration of one or more effects of prevention of complication; verbalizes that family did not take action to reduce risk factors for progression of illness and sequelae.

Memory, Impaired
Definition
The state in which an individual experiences the inability to remember or recall bits of information or behavioral skills. Impaired memory may be attributed to pathophysiologic or situational causes that are either temporary or permanent.

Defining Characteristics
Major: Observed or reported experiences of forgetting; inability to determine whether a behavior was performed; inability to learn or retain new skills or information; inability to perform a previously learned skill; inability to recall factual information; inability to recall recent or past events.

Minor: Forgets to perform a behavior at a scheduled time.

Noncompliance
Definition
A person's informed decision not to adhere to a therapeutic recommendation.

Defining Characteristics
Behavior indicative of failure to adhere (by direct observation or by statements of patient or significant others)*; objective tests (physiologic measures, detection of markers); evidence of development of complications; evidence of exacerbation of symptoms; failure to keep appointments; failure to progress.

---
*Critical

Nutrition, Altered: More Than Body Requirements
Definition
The state in which an individual is experiencing an intake of nutrients that exceeds metabolic needs.

Defining Characteristics
Weight 10% over ideal for height and frame; weight 20% over ideal for height and frame*; triceps skin fold greater than 15 mm in men, 25 mm in women*; sedentary activity level; reported or observed dysfunctional eating pattern: pairing food with other activities; concentrating food intake at the end of day; eating in response to external cues such as time of day, social situation; eating in response to internal cues other than hunger, e.g., anxiety.

---
*Critical

Nutrition, Altered: Less Than Body Requirements
Definition
The state in which an individual experiences an intake of nutrients insufficient to meet metabolic needs.

Defining Characteristics
Loss of weight with adequate food intake; body weight 20% or more under ideal; reported inadequate food intake less than recommended daily allowance (RDA); weakness of muscles required for swallowing or mastication; reported or evidence of lack of food; aversion to eating; reported altered taste sensation; satiety immediately after ingesting food; abdominal pain with or without pathology; sore, inflamed buccal cavity; capillary fragility; abdominal cramping; diarrhea and/or steatorrhea; hyperactive bowel sounds; lack of interest in food; perceived inability to ingest food; pale conjunctival and mucous membranes; poor muscle tone; excessive loss of hair; lack of information, misinformation; misconceptions.

Oral Mucous Membrane, Altered
Definition
The state in which an individual experiences disruptions in the tissue layers of the oral cavity.

Defining Characteristics
Oral pain/discomfort; coated tongue; xerostomia (dry mouth); stomatitis; oral lesions or ulcers; lack of or decreased salivation; leukoplakia; edema; hyperemia; oral plaque; desquamation; vesicles; hemorrhagic gingivitis, carious teeth; halitosis.

Pain
Definition
A state in which an individual experiences and reports the presence of severe discomfort or an uncomfortable sensation.

Defining Characteristics

Subjective: Communication (verbal or coded) of pain descriptors.

Objective: Guarded behavior, protective; self-focusing; narrowed focus (altered time perception, withdrawal from social contact, impaired thought process); distraction behavior (moaning, crying, pacing, seeking out other people and/or activities, restlessness); facial mask of pain (eyes lack luster, beaten look, fixed or scattered movement, grimace); alteration in muscle tone (may span from listless to rigid); autonomic responses not seen in chronic stable pain (diaphoresis, blood pressure and pulse change, pupillary dilation, increased or decreased respiratory rate).

Pain, Chronic
Definition
A state in which the individual experiences pain that continues for more than 6 months in duration.

Defining Characteristics
Major: Verbal report or observed evidence of pain experienced for more than 6 months.

Minor: Fear of reinjury; physical and social withdrawal; altered ability to continue previous activities; anorexia; weight changes; changes in sleep patterns; facial mask of pain; guarded movement.

Parenting, Risk for Altered
Definition
The state in which a nurturing figure(s) is at risk to experience an inability to create an environment that promotes the optimal growth and development of another human being.[†]

Defining Characteristics
Presence of risk factors such as: Lack of parental attachment behaviors; inappropriate visual, tactile, auditory stimulation; negative identification of infant/child's characteristics; negative attachment of meanings to infant/child's characteristics; constant verbalization of disappointment in gender or physical characteristics of the infant/child; verbalization of resentment toward the infant/child; verbalization of role inadequacy; inattentive to infant/child's needs*; verbal disgust at body functions of infant/child; noncompliance with health appointments for self and/or infant/child; inappropriate caretaking behaviors (toilet training, sleep/rest, feeding)*; inappropriate or inconsistent discipline practices; frequent accidents; frequent illness; growth and development lag in the child; history of child abuse or abandonment by primary caretaker*; verbalizes desire to have child call him/herself by first name versus traditional cultural tendencies; child receives care from multiple caretakers without consideration for the needs of the infant/child; compulsively seeking role approval from others.

---

*Critical

[†]It is important to state as a preface to this diagnosis that adjustment to parenting in general is a normal maturational process that elicits nursing behaviors of prevention of potential problems and health promotion.

Peripheral Neurovascular Dysfunction, Risk for
Definition
A state in which an individual is at risk of experiencing a disruption in circulation, sensation, or motion of an extremity.

Risk Factors
Fractures; mechanical compression, e.g., tourniquet, cast, knee dressing or restraint; orthopedic surgery; trauma; immobilization; burns; vascular obstruction.

Perioperative Positioning Injury, Risk for
Definition
A state in which the client is at risk for injury as a result of the environmental conditions found in the perioperative setting.

Risk Factors
Disorientation; immobilization, muscle weakness; sensory/perceptual disturbance due to anesthesia; obesity; emaciation; edema.

Personal Identity Disturbance
Definition
Inability to distinguish between self and nonself.

Defining Characteristics
To be developed.

Physical Mobility, Impaired
Definition
A state in which the individual experiences a limitation of ability for independent physical movement.

Defining Characteristics
Inability to purposefully move within the physical environment, including bed mobility, transfer, and ambula-

tion; reluctance to attempt movement; limited range of motion; decreased muscle strength, control and/or mass; imposed restrictions of movement, including mechanical, medical protocol; impaired coordination.

Post-Trauma Response
Definition
The state of an individual's experiencing a sustained painful response to an overwhelming traumatic event(s).

Defining Characteristics
Major: Re-experience of the traumatic event, which may be identified in cognitive, affective, and/or sensory motor activities (flashbacks, intrusive thoughts, repetitive dreams or nightmares, excessive verbalization of the traumatic event, verbalization of survival guilt or guilt about behavior required for survival).

Minor: Psychic/emotional numbness (impaired interpretation of reality, confusion, dissociation or amnesia, vagueness about traumatic event, constricted affect); altered lifestyle (self-destructiveness, such as substance abuse, suicide attempt, or other acting out behavior, difficulty with interpersonal relationship, development of phobia regarding trauma, poor impulse control/irritability and explosiveness).

Powerlessness
Definition
Perception that one's own actions will not significantly affect an outcome; a perceived lack of control over a current situation or immediate happening.

Defining Characteristics
Severe: Verbal expressions of having no control or influence over situation; verbal expressions of having no control or influence over outcome; verbal expressions of having no control over self-care; depression over physical deterioration that occurs despite patient compliance with regimens; apathy.

Moderate: Nonparticipation in care or decision making when opportunities are provided; expressions of dissatisfaction and frustration over inability to perform previous tasks and/or activities; does not monitor progress; expression of doubt regarding role performance; reluctance to express true feelings; fearing alienation from caregivers; passivity; inability to seek information regarding care; dependence on others that may result in irritability, resentment, anger, and guilt; does not defend self-care practices when challenged.

Low: Expressions of uncertainty about fluctuating energy levels; passivity.

Protection, Altered
Definition
The state in which an individual experiences a decrease in the ability to guard the self from internal or external threats such as illness or injury.

Defining Characteristics
Major: Deficient immunity; impaired healing; altered clotting; maladaptive stress response; neurosensory alteration.

Minor: Chilling; perspiring; dyspnea; cough; itching; restlessness; insomnia; fatigue; anorexia; weakness; immobility; disorientation; pressure sores.

Relocation Stress Syndrome
Definition
Physiologic and/or psychosocial disturbances as a result of transfer from one environment to another.

Defining Characteristics
Major: Change in environment/location; anxiety; apprehension; increased confusion (elderly population); depression; loneliness.

Minor: Verbalization of unwillingness to relocate; sleep disturbance; change in eating habits; dependency; gastrointestinal disturbances; increased verbalization of needs; insecurity; lack of trust; restlessness; sad affect; unfavorable comparison of post/pre-transfer staff; verbalization of being concerned/upset about transfer; vigilance; weight change; withdrawal.

Role Conflict, Parental
Definition
The state in which a parent experiences role confusion and conflict in response to crisis.

Defining Characteristics
Major: Parent(s) expresses concerns/feelings of inadequacy to provide for child's physical and emotional needs during hospitalization or in the home; demonstrated disruption in caretaking routines; parent(s) expresses concerns about changes in parental role, family functioning, family communication, family health.

Minor: Expresses concern about perceived loss of control over decisions relating to the child; reluctant to participate in usual caretaking activities even with encouragement and support; verbalizes, demonstrates feelings of guilt, anger, fear, anxiety and/or frustrations about effect of child's illness on family process.

Role Performance, Altered
Definition
Disruption in the way one perceives one's role performance.

Defining Characteristics
Change in self-perception of role; denial of role; change in others' perception of role; conflict in roles; change in physical capacity to resume role; lack of knowledge of role; change in usual patterns of responsibility.

Self-Care Deficit, Feeding
Definition
A state in which the individual experiences an impaired ability to perform or complete feeding activities for oneself.

Defining Characteristics
Inability to bring food from a receptacle to the mouth.

Self-Care Deficit, Bathing/Hygiene
Definition
A state in which the individual experiences an impaired ability to perform or complete bathing/hygiene activities for oneself.

Defining Characteristics
Inability to wash body or body parts*: inability to obtain or get to water source; inability to regulate water temperature or flow.

---

*Critical

Self-Care Deficit, Dressing/Grooming
Definition
A state in which the individual experiences an impaired ability to perform or complete dressing and grooming activities for oneself.

Defining Characteristics
Impaired ability to put on or take off necessary items of clothing*; impaired ability to obtain or replace articles of clothing; impaired ability to fasten clothing; inability to maintain appearance at a satisfactory level.

---

*Critical

Self-Care Deficit, Toileting
Definition
A state in which the individual experiences an impaired ability to perform or complete toileting activities for oneself.

Defining Characteristics
Unable to get to toilet or commode*; unable to sit on or rise from toilet or commode*; unable to manipulate clothing for toileting*; unable to carry out proper toilet hygiene*; unable to flush toilet or commode.

---

*Critical

Self-Esteem Disturbance
Definition
Negative self-evaluation/feelings about self or self-capabilities, which may be directly or indirectly expressed.

Defining Characteristics
Self-negating verbalization; expressions of shame/guilt; evaluates self as unable to deal with events; rationalizes away/rejects positive feedback and exaggerates negative feedback about self; hesitant to try new things/situations; denial of problems obvious to others; projection of blame/responsibility for problems; rationalizing personal failures.

Self-Esteem, Chronic Low
Definition
Long-standing negative self-evaluation/feelings about self or self-capabilities.

Defining Characteristics
Major: Long-standing or chronic: self-negating verbalization; expressions of shame/guilt; evaluates self as unable to deal with events; rationalizes away/rejects positive feedback and exaggerates negative feedback about self; hesitant to try new things/situations.

Minor: Frequent lack of success in work or other life events; overly conforming, dependent on others' opinions; lack of eye contact; nonassertive/passive; indecisive; excessively seeks reassurance.

Self-Esteem, Situational Low
Definition
Negative self-evaluation/feelings about self that develop in response to a loss or change in an individual who previously had a positive self-evaluation.

Defining Characteristics
Major: Episodic occurrence of negative self-appraisal in response to life events in a person with a previous positive self-evaluation; verbalization of negative feelings about the self (helplessness, uselessness).

Minor: Self-negating verbalizations; expressions of shame/guilt; evaluates self as unable to handle situations/events; difficulty making decisions.

Sensory/Perceptual Alterations
Definition
A state in which an individual experiences a change in the amount or patterning of oncoming stimuli accompanied by a diminished, exaggerated, distorted, or impaired response to such stimuli.

Defining Characteristics
Disoriented in time, in place, or with persons; altered abstraction; altered conceptualization; change in problem-solving abilities; reported or measured change in sensory acuity; change in behavior pattern; anxiety; apathy; change in usual response to stimuli; indication of body-image alteration; restlessness; irritability; altered communication patterns.

Other Possible Characteristics
Complaints of fatigue; alteration in posture; change in muscular tension; inappropriate responses; hallucinations.

Sexual Dysfunction
Definition
The state in which an individual experiences a change in sexual function that is viewed as unsatisfying, unrewarding, inadequate.

Defining Characteristics
Verbalization of problem; alterations in achieving perceived sex role; actual or perceived limitation imposed by disease and/or therapy; conflicts involving values; alteration in achieving sexual satisfaction; inability to achieve desired satisfaction; seeking confirmation of desirability; alteration in relationship with significant other; change of interest in self and others.

Sexuality Patterns, Altered
Definition
The state in which an individual expresses concern regarding his/her sexuality.

Defining Characteristics
Major: Reported difficulties, limitations, or changes in sexual behaviors or activities.

Skin Integrity, Impaired
Definition
A state in which the individual's skin is adversely altered.

Defining Characteristics
Disruption of skin surface; destruction of skin layers; invasion of body structures.

Skin Integrity, Risk for Impaired
Definition
A state in which the individual's skin is at risk of being adversely altered.

Defining Characteristics
Presence of risk factors such as:
External (environmental): Hypothermia or hyperthermia; chemical substance; mechanical factors (shearing forces, pressure, restraint); radiation; physical immobilization; excretions/secretions; humidity.

Internal (somatic): Medication; alterations in nutritional state (obesity, emaciation); altered metabolic state; altered circulation; altered sensation; altered pigmentation; skeletal prominence; developmental factors; alterations in skin turgor (change in elasticity); psychogenic; immunologic.

Sleep Pattern Disturbance
Definition
Disruption of sleep time causes discomfort or interferes with desired lifestyle.

Defining Characteristics
Verbal complaints of difficulty falling asleep*; awakening earlier or later than desired*; interrupted sleep*; verbal complaints of not feeling well-rested*; changes in behavior and performance (increasing irritability, restlessness, disorientation, lethargy, listlessness); physical signs (mild fleeting nystagmus, slight hand tremor, ptosis of eyelid, expressionless face, dark circles under eyes, frequent yawning, changes in posture); thick speech with mispronunciation and incorrect words.

*Critical

Social Interaction, Impaired
Definition
The state in which an individual participates in an insufficient or excessive quantity or ineffective quality of social exchange.

Defining Characteristics
Major: Verbalized or observed discomfort in social situations: verbalized or observed inability to receive or communicate a satisfying sense of belonging, caring, interest, or shared history; observed use of unsuccessful social interaction behaviors; dysfunctional interaction with peers, family and/or others.

Minor: Family report of change of style or pattern of interaction.

Spiritual Distress
Definition
Disruption in the life principle which pervades a person's entire being and which integrates and transcends one's biologic and psychosocial nature.

Defining Characteristics
Expresses concern with meaning of life/death and/or belief systems*; anger toward God; questions meaning of suffering; verbalizes inner conflict about beliefs; verbalizes concern about relationship with deity; questions meaning of own existence; unable to participate in usual religious practices; seeks spiritual assistance; questions moral/ethical implications of therapeutic regimen; gallows humor; displacement of anger toward religious representatives; description of nightmares/sleep disturbances; alteration in behavior/mood evidenced by anger, crying, withdrawal, preoccupation, anxiety, hostility, apathy, and so forth.

---

*Critical

Swallowing, Impaired
Definition
The state in which an individual has decreased ability to voluntarily pass fluids and/or solids from the mouth to the stomach.

Defining Characteristics
Major: Observed evidence of difficulty in swallowing, e.g., stasis of food in oral cavity, coughing/choking.

Minor: Evidence of aspiration.

Thermoregulation, Ineffective
Definition
The state in which the individual's body temperature fluctuates between hypothermia and hyperthermia.

Defining Characteristics
Major: Fluctuations in body temperature above or below the normal range. See also major and minor characteristics present in hypothermia and hyperthermia.

Thought Processes, Altered
Definition
A state in which an individual experiences a disruption in cognitive operations and activities.

Defining Characteristics
Accurate interpretation of environment; cognitive dissonance; distractibility; memory deficit/problems; egocentricity; hypervigilance or hypovigilance.

Other Possible Characteristics
Inappropriate nonreality-based thinking.

Tissue Integrity, Impaired
Definition
A state in which an individual experiences damage to mucous membrane, corneal, integumentary, or subcutaneous tissue.

Defining Characteristics
Major: Damaged or destroyed tissue (cornea, mucous membrane, integumentary, or subcutaneous).

Tissue Perfusion, Altered
Definition
The state in which an individual experiences a decrease in nutrition and oxygenation at the cellular level that is due to a deficit in capillary blood supply.

Defining Characteristics

	Chances that characteristics will be present given diagnosis	Estimated sensitivities and specificities. Chances that characteristic will not be explained by any other diagnosis
Skin temperature, cold extremities	High	Low
Skin color dependent blue or purple	Moderate	Low
Pale on elevation, color does not return on lowering of leg*	High	High
Diminished arterial pulsations*	High	High
Skin quality: Shining	High	Low
Lack of lanugo	High	Moderate
Round scars covered with atrophied skin		
Gangrene	Low	High
Slow-growing, dry brittle nails	High	Moderate
Claudication	Moderate	High
Blood pressure changes in extremities		
Bruits	Moderate	Moderate
Slow healing of lesions	High	Low

*Critical

Trauma, Risk for

Definition

Accentuated risk of accidental tissue injury, e.g., wound, burn, fracture.

Defining Characteristics

Presence of risk factors such as:

Internal (individual): Weakness; poor vision; balancing difficulties; reduced temperature and/or tactile sensation; reduced large or small muscle coordination; reduced hand-eye coordination; lack of safety education; lack of safety precautions; insufficient finances to purchase safety equipment or effect repairs; cognitive or emotional difficulties; history of previous trauma.

External (environmental): Slippery floors, e.g., wet or highly waxed; snow or ice collected on stairs, walkways; unanchored rugs; bathtub without hand grip or antislip equipment; use of unsteady ladders or chairs; entering unlighted rooms; unsturdy or absent stair rails; unanchored electric wires; litter or liquid spills on floors or stairways; high beds; children playing without gates at the top of the stairs; obstructed passageways; unsafe window protection in homes with young children; inappropriate call-for-aid mechanisms for bed-resting client; pot handles facing toward front of stove; bathing in very hot water, e.g., unsupervised bathing of young children; potential igniting gas leaks; delayed lighting of gas burner or oven; experimenting with chemical or gasoline; unscreened fires or heaters; wearing plastic apron or flowing clothes around open flame; children playing with matches, candles, cigarettes; inadequately stored combustibles or corrosives, e.g., matches, oily rags, lye; highly flammable children's toys or clothing; overloaded fuse boxes; contact with rapidly moving machinery, industrial belts or pulleys; sliding on coarse bed linen or struggling within bed restraints; faulty electrical plugs, frayed wires, or defective appliances; contact with acids or alkalies; playing with fireworks or gunpowder; contact with intense cold; overexposure to sun, sun lamps, radiotherapy; use of cracked dishware or glasses; knives stored uncovered; guns or ammunition stored unlocked; large icicles hanging from the roof; exposure to dangerous machinery; children playing with sharp-edged toys; high-crime neighborhood and vulnerable clients; driving a mechanically unsafe vehicle; driving after partaking of alcoholic beverages or drugs; driving at excessive speeds; driving without necessary visual aids; children riding unrestrained in the front seat in car; smoking in bed or near oxygen; overloaded electrical outlets; grease waste collected on stoves; use of thin or worn potholders or misuse of necessary headgear for motorized cyclists or young children carried on adult bicycles; unsafe road or road-crossing conditions; play or work near vehicle pathways, e.g., driveways, laneways, railroad tracks; nonuse or misuse of seat restraints.

Unilateral Neglect

Definition

A state in which an individual is perceptually unaware of, and inattentive to, one side of the body.

Defining Characteristics

Major: Consistent inattention to stimuli on an affected side.

Minor: Inadequate self-care; positioning and/or safety precautions in regard to the affected side; does not look toward affected side; leaves food on plate on the affected side.

Urinary Elimination, Altered

Definition

The state in which the individual experiences a disturbance in urine elimination.

Defining Characteristics

Dysuria; frequency; hesitancy; incontinence; nocturia; retention; urgency.

Urinary Retention

Definition

The state in which the individual experiences incomplete emptying of the bladder.

Defining Characteristics

Major: Bladder distention; small, frequent voiding or absence of urine output.

Minor: Sensation of bladder fullness; dribbling; residual urine; dysuria; overflow incontinence.

Ventilation, Inability to Sustain Spontaneous

Definition

A state in which the response pattern of decreased energy reserves results in an individual's inability to maintain breathing adequate to support life.

Defining Characteristics

Major: Dyspnea; increased metabolic rate.

Minor: Increased restlessness; apprehension; increased use of accessory muscles; decreased tidal volume; increased heart rate, decreased pO_2; increased pCO_2; decreased cooperation; decreased SaO_2.

Verbal Communication, Impaired

Definition

The state in which an individual experiences a decreased or absent ability to use or understand language in human interaction.

Defining Characteristics

Unable to speak dominant language*; speaks or verbalizes with difficulty*; does not or cannot speak*; stuttering; slurring; difficulty forming words or sentences; difficulty expressing thoughts verbally; inappropriate verbalization; dyspnea; disorientation.

---

*Critical

Overview of Functional Health Patterns

Health Perception/Health Management:
Description of health (usual and present); relevance of health to activities; preventive measures; immunizations; general health care behavior; family history; allergies. Previous hospitalizations; expectations of this hospitalization. Description of illness (onset, course, treatment); potential self-care problems.

Nutritional/Metabolic: Usual food and fluid intake; daily eating times. Appetite; food restrictions, preferences or allergies; food supplements. Recent weight change. Swallowing, chewing, or eating problems. Skin lesions and general ability to heal; condition of skin, hair, nails, mucous membranes, and teeth. Temperature, pulse, respirations; height and weight.

Elimination: Bowel: Usual time, frequency, color, consistency; assistive devices (laxatives, suppositories, enemas); constipation; diarrhea. Bladder: Usual frequency; problems with dysuria or polyuria, assistive devices. Skin: Condition; color; temperature; turgor; lesions; edema; pruritus.

Activity/Exercise: Usual exercise activities; leisure/recreation patterns; limitations in activities of daily living.

Sleep: Usual sleep routine; sleep pattern; sleep aids.

Cognitive/Perceptual: Sensory adequacy: Hearing; sight; touch. Prosthetic devices; problems with vertigo; heat or cold sensitivity. Pain. Ability to use language; understanding; memory.

Self-Perception: Self-description; effects of illness on self. Perception: Body image; identity; self-esteem. Posture; eye contact; voice and speech patterns.

Role/Relationship: Life roles and responsibilities; satisfaction/dissatisfaction in family, work, and social relationships.

Sexuality/Reproductive: Sexuality patterns and satisfaction/dissatisfaction with. Reproductive stage (female): Pre/post menopausal.

Coping/Stress Tolerance: General coping; stress tolerance; stress reduction behaviors. Support systems. Ability to manage situation.

Value/Belief: Values, goals, beliefs that are basis for decisions; values/belief conflict.

Modified from Gordon M: *Manual of nursing diagnoses 1995–1996,* St Louis, 1995, Mosby.

Nursing History: Functional Health Pattern Format

Demographic Data

Name, address, age, occupation

Important Medical Information

Past health history
Medications
Surgery or other treatments

Functional Health Patterns

Health perception/health management pattern
1. Reason for visit?
2. General state of health?
3. Any colds in past year?
4. Most important things done to keep healthy? Breast self-examination? Testicular self-examination? Other routine screening?
5. Health compliance problems?
6. Cause of illness? Action taken? Results?
7. Things important to you while here?
8. Family health history?
9. Illness and injury risk factors: use of cigarettes, alcohol, drugs?
10. Allergies? Immunizations?

Nutritional/metabolic pattern
1. Typical daily food intake (describe)? Supplements?
2. Typical daily fluid intake (describe)?
3. Weight loss/gain (amount, time span)?
4. Desired weight?
5. Appetite?
6. Food or eating: Discomfort? Diet restrictions?
7. Appetite?
8. Heal well or poorly?
9. Skin problems: Lesions? Dryness?
10. Dental problems?
11. Change in appetite with anxiety?
12. Food preferences?
13. Food allergies?

Elimination pattern
1. Bowel elimination pattern (describe): Frequency? Character? Discomfort? Laxatives? Enemas?
2. Urinary elimination pattern (describe): Frequency? Problem in control? Diuretics?
3. Any external devices?
4. Excess perspiration? Odor problems? Itching?

Activity/exercise pattern
1. Sufficient energy for desired/required activities?
2. Exercise pattern? Type? Regularity?
3. Spare time (leisure) activities?

4. Dyspnea? Chest pain? Palpitations? Stiffness? Aching? Weakness?
5. Perceived ability for (code for level):

Feeding _____
Grooming _____
Bathing _____
General mobility _____
Toileting _____
Cooking _____
Bed mobility _____
Home maintenance _____
Dressing _____
Shopping _____

Functional levels code

Level 0:   Full self-care
Level I: Requires use of equipment or device
Level II: Requires assistance or supervision from another person
Level III: Is dependent and does not participate

Sleep/rest pattern

1. Generally rested and ready for daily activities after sleep?
2. Sleep onset problems? Aids? Dreams (nightmares)? Early awakening?
3. Usual sleep rituals?
4. Usual sleep pattern?

Cognitive/perceptual pattern

1. Hearing difficulty? Aid?
2. Vision? Wear glasses? Last checked?
3. Any change in taste? Any change in smell?
4. Any recent change in memory?
5. Easiest way to learn things?
6. Any discomfort? Pain? How managed?
7. Ability to communicate?
8. Understanding of illness?
9. Understanding of treatments?

Self-perception/self-concept pattern

1. Self-description? Self-perception?
2. Effect of illness on self-image?
3. Relieving factors?

Role/relationship pattern

1. Live alone? Family? Family structure diagram?
2. Difficult family problems?
3. Family problem solving?
4. Family depend on you for things? How managing?
5. Family/others feelings about illness/hospitalization?
6. Problems with children? Difficulty handling?
7. Belong to social groups? Close friends? Feel lonely (frequency)?
8. Work satisfaction (school)? Income sufficient for needs?
9. Feel part of or isolated from neighborhood where living?

Sexuality/reproductive pattern

1. Any changes or problems in sexual relations?
2. Effect of illness?
3. Use of contraceptives? Problems?
4. When menstruation started? Last menstrual period? Menstrual problems? Para? Gravida?
5. Effect of present condition or treatment on sexuality?
6. Sexually transmitted diseases?

Coping/stress-tolerance pattern

1. Tense a lot of the time? What helps? Use any medicines, drugs, alcohol?
2. Have someone to confide in? Available to you now?
3. Recent life changes?
4. Problem-solving techniques? Effective?

Value/belief pattern

1. Satisfied with life?
2. Religion important in your life?
3. Conflict between treatment and beliefs?
4. Cultural beliefs that impact this admission?

Other

1. Other important issues?
2. Questions?

Modified from Fuller J, Schaller-Ayers J: *Health assessment: a nursing approach,* ed 2, New York, 1994, JB Lippincott.

Comprehensive Physical Examination

1. **General Survey**
   a. Observe general state of health (client is seated):
   Body features
   State of consciousness and arousal
   Speech
   Body movements
   Physical signs
   Nutritional status
   Stature

2. **Vital Signs**
   a. Record vital signs:
   Blood pressure
   Radial pulse
   Respiration
   b. Record height and weight

3. **Integumentary System**
   a. Inspect and palpate skin for the following:
   Color
   Lesions
   Scars
   Bruises
   Edema
   Moisture
   Texture
   Temperature
   Turgor
   Vascularity

   b. Inspect and palpate nails for the following:
   Color
   Lesions
   Size
   Flexibility
   Shape
   Angle

4. **Head and Neck**
   a. Inspect and palpate head for the following:
   Shape and symmetry of skull
   Masses
   Tenderness
   Hair
   Scalp
   Skin
   Temporal arteries
   Temporomandibular joint
   Sensory (cranial nerve [CN] V, light touch and pain)
   Motor (CN VII, shows teeth, purses lips, raises eyebrows)
   Looking up and wrinkling forehead (CN VII)
   Raise shoulders against resistance (CN XI)
   b. Inspect and palpate eyes for the following:
   Visual acuity
   Eyebrows
   Position and movement of eyelids
   Visual fields

Extraocular movements (CN III, IV, VI)
Cornea, sclera, conjunctiva
Pupillary response
Red reflex
Eyeball tension

c. Inspect and palpate ears for the following:
Placement
Pinna
Auditory acuity (Weber or Rinne, whispered voice, ticking watch)
Mastoid process
Auditory canal
Tympanic membrane

d. Inspect and palpate nose and sinuses for the following:
External nose
  Shape
  Blockage
Internal nose
  Patency of nasal passages
  Shape
  Turbinates/polyps
  Discharge
Frontal and maxillary sinuses

e. Inspect and palpate mouth for the following:
Lips (symmetry, lesions, color)
Buccal mucosa (Stensen's and Wharton's ducts)
Teeth (absent, state of repair, color)
Gums
Tongue for strength (asymmetry, ability to stick out tongue, side to side, fasciculations)
Palates
Tonsils and pillars
Uvular elevation (CN IX)
Posterior pharynx
Gag reflex (CN X)
Jaw strength (CN XI)
Moisture
Color
Floor of mouth

f. Inspect and palpate (occasionally auscultate) neck for the following:
Skin (vascularity and visible pulsations)
Symmetry
Postural alignment
Range of motion
Pulses (carotid)
Midline structure (trachea, thyroid gland, and cartilage)
Lymph nodes (preauricular, postauricular, occipital, mandibular, tonsillar, submental, anterior and posterior cervical, infraclavicular, supraclavicular)

5. **Inspect Neurologic Status:**
  a. Motor status observations:
   Gait
   Toe walk
   Heel walk
   Drift
  b. Coordination
   Finger to nose
   Romberg's sign
  c. Spine (scoliosis)

6. **Extremities**
  a. Observe:
   Size and shape
   Symmetry
   Deformity
   Involuntary movements
  b. Inspect and palpate arms, fingers, wrists, elbows, and shoulders for:
   Strength
   Range of motion
   Crepitus
   Joint pain
   Swelling
   Fluid
  c. Test reflexes:
   Biceps
   Triceps
   Brachioradialis
   Patellar
   Achilles
   Plantar
  d. Inspect and palpate legs for:
   Strength of hips
   Edema
   Hair distribution
   Pulses (dorsalis pedis, posterior tibialis)
   Joint pain
   Fluid

7. **Posterior Thorax**
  a. Inspect for:
   Muscular development
   Respiratory movement
   Approximation of A-P diameter
  b. Palpate for:
   Symmetry of respiratory movement
   CVA tenderness
   Spinous processes
   Tumors or swelling
   Tactile fremitus
  c. Percuss for pulmonary resonance
  d. Auscultate breath sounds

8. **Anterior Thorax**
   a. Assess breasts for: (client is upright)
      Configuration
      Symmetry
      Dimpling of skin
      Rash
   b. Assess nipples for:
      Direction
      Inversion
      Retraction
   c. Initiate teaching or review of breast self-examination
   d. Inspect chest for:
      PMI
      Other precordial pulsations
   e. Palpate chest for:
      Thrills
      Lifts
      Heaves
      Tenderness over precordium
   f. Inspect neck for:
      Venous distention
      Pulsations
      Waves
   g. Palpate axillae
   h. Inspect palpate, check breasts for discharge (client is supine)
   i. Complete teaching of breast self-examination
   j. Auscultate for:
      Heart rate and rhythm
      Character of S_1 and S_2
      S_1 and S_2 in aortic, pulmonic, Erb's point, tricuspid, and mitral areas
      Bruits at carotid, epigastrium
      Breath sounds

9. **Abdomen**
   a. Inspect for:
      Scars
      Shape
      Symmetry
      Bulging
      Muscular development
      Position and condition of umbilicus,
      Movements (respiratory, pulsations, presence of peristaltic waves)
   b. Auscultate for:
      Bowel sounds
      Abdominal aortic and femoral bruits
   c. Percuss for:
      Border of liver
      All quadrants for tumors or masses

   d. Palpate:
      Confirm positive findings
      Liver (size, surface contour, tenderness)
      Spleen, kidneys (size, contour, consistency, tenderness, mobility)
      Urinary bladder (distention)
      Femoral pulses
      Inguinofemoral nodes

10. **Completion of Examination of Extremities**
    a. Observe the following:
       Range of motion of hips, ankles, feet
       Crepitus
       Joint pain
       Swelling
       Fluid
       Muscle development
       Coordination (heel to shin)
       Homans' sign
       Proprioception (position sense of great toe)

11. **Male Genitalia***
    a. Inspect penis and note:
       Hair distribution
       Prepuce
       Glans
       Urethral meatus
       Scars
       Ulcers
       Eruptions
       Structural alterations
    b. Inspect skin of scrotum
    c. Palpate for:
       Descended testes
       Masses
       Pain
    d. Inspect epidermis of perineum, rectum

12. **Female Genitalia**
    a. Inspect:
       Hair distribution
       Mons pubis
       Labia (minora and majora)
       Urethral meatus
       Bartholin's, urethral, Skene's glands (may also be palpated, if indicated)
       Introitus
    b. Assess for presence of cystocele, rectocele, prolapse (client bears down)
    c. Inspect epidermis of perineum, rectum

---

*If the nurse has the appropriate education, the prostate gland examination of men and the speculum and bimanual examination of women should be performed after this inspection.

Diagnostic Labels Grouped by Functional Health Patterns, 1995–1996

Health Perception/Health Management Pattern

Altered Health Maintenance
Ineffective Management of Therapeutic Regimen
Noncompliance (Specify)
Health-Seeking Behaviors (Specify)
Risk for Infection
Risk for Injury (Trauma)
Risk for Poisoning
Risk for Suffocation
Altered Protection
Ineffective Management of Therapeutic Regimen: Families*
Ineffective Management of Therapeutic Regimen: Community*
Ineffective Management of Therapeutic Regimen: Individual*
Risk for Perioperative Positioning Injury*
Energy Field Disturbance*

Nutritional/Metabolic Pattern

Altered Nutrition: Risk for More than Body Requirements
Altered Nutrition: More than Body Requirements
Altered Nutrition: Less than Body Requirements
Ineffective Breastfeeding

Effective Breastfeeding
Interrupted Breastfeeding
Ineffective Infant Feeding Pattern
Risk for Aspiration
Impaired Swallowing
Altered Oral Mucous Membrane
Risk for Fluid Volume Deficit
Fluid Volume Deficit
Fluid Volume Excess
Risk for Impaired Skin Integrity
Impaired Skin Integrity
Impaired Tissue Integrity
Risk for Altered Body Temperature
Ineffective Thermoregulation
Hyperthermia
Hypothermia

Elimination Pattern

Constipation
Colonic Constipation
Perceived Constipation
Diarrhea
Bowel Incontinence
Altered Urinary Elimination Patterns
Functional Incontinence
Reflex Incontinence
Stress Incontinence
Urge Incontinence
Total Incontinence
Urinary Retention

Modified from *NANDA nursing diagnosis: definitions and classifications 1995–1996*, North American Nursing Diagnosis Association; and Gordon M: *Manual of nursing diagnoses 1995–1996*, St Louis, 1995, Mosby.

Activity/Exercise Pattern

Risk for Activity Intolerance
Activity Intolerance (Specify Level)
Fatigue
Impaired Physical Mobility (Specify Level)
Risk for Disuse Syndrome
Total Self-Care Deficit (Specify Level)
Self Care Deficit, Bathing/Hygiene (Specify Level)
Self Care Deficit, Dressing/Grooming (Specify Level)
Self Care Deficit, Feeding (Specify Level)
Self Care Deficit, Toileting (Specify Level)
Diversional Activity Deficit
Impaired Home Maintenance Management (Mild, Moderate, Severe, High Risk, Chronic)
Dysfunctional Ventilatory Weaning Response (DVWR)
Inability to Sustain Spontaneous Ventilation
Ineffective Airway Clearance
Ineffective Breathing Pattern
Impaired Gas Exchange
Decreased Cardiac Output
Altered Tissue Perfusion (Specify)
Dysreflexia
Risk for Peripheral Neurovascular Dysfunction
Altered Growth and Development
Risk for Disorganized Infant Behavior*
Disorganized Infant Behavior*
Potential for Enhanced Organized Infant Behavior*

Sleep/Rest Pattern

Sleep Pattern Disturbance

Cognitive/Perceptual Pattern

Pain
Chronic Pain
Sensory/Perceptual Alterations
Unilateral Neglect
Knowledge Deficit (Specify)
Impaired Thought Processes
Decisional Conflict (Specify)
Decreased Adaptive Capacity: Intracranial*
Impaired Environmental Interpretation Syndrome*
Acute Confusion*
Chronic Confusion*
Impaired Memory*

Self-Perception/Self-Concept Pattern

Fear (Specify Focus)
Anxiety
Hopelessness
Powerlessness (Severe, Low, Moderate)

Self-Esteem Disturbance
Chronic Low Self-Esteem
Situational Low Self-Esteem
Body Image Disturbance
Risk for Self-Mutilation
Personal Identity Disturbance
Risk for Loneliness*

Role/Relationship Pattern

Anticipatory Grieving
Dysfunctional Grieving
Disturbance in Role Performance
Social Isolation
Impaired Social Interaction
Relocation Stress Syndrome
Altered Family Processes
Risk for Altered Parenting
Altered Parenting
Parental Role Conflict
Caregiver Role Strain
Risk for Caregiver Role Strain
Impaired Verbal Communication
Risk for Violence
Risk for Altered Parent/Infant/Child Relationship*
Altered Family Processes: Alcoholism*

Sexuality/Reproductive Pattern

Sexual Dysfunction (Specify Type)
Altered Sexuality Patterns
Rape-Trauma Syndrome
Rape-Trauma Syndrome: Compound Reaction
Rape-Trauma Syndrome: Silent Reaction

Coping/Stress Tolerance Pattern

Ineffective Coping (Individual)
Defensive Coping
Ineffective Denial
Impaired Adjustment
Post-Trauma Response
Family Coping: Potential for Growth
Ineffective Family Coping: Compromised
Ineffective Family Coping: Disabling
Potential for Enhanced Community Coping*
Ineffective Community Coping*

Value/Belief Pattern

Spiritual Distress (Distress of the Human Spirit)
Potential for Enhanced Spiritual Well-being*

---

*New diagnoses added in 1995.

References

1. *Nursing: a social policy statement,* Kansas City, Mo, 1985, American Nurses Association.
2. Gordon M: *Nursing diagnosis: process and application,* ed 3, St. Louis, 1994, Mosby.
3. North American Nursing Diagnosis Association: *NANDA nursing diagnoses: definitions and classification 1995–1996,* Philadelphia, 1994, NANDA.
4. Lunney M: Accuracy of nursing diagnoses: concept development, *Nursing Diagnosis* 1:12, Jan/Mar. 1990.
5. Carpenito L: *Nursing diagnosis: application to clinical practice,* ed 6, Philadelphia, 1995, JB Lippincott.
6. Briody ME and others: Toward further understanding of nursing diagnosis, an interpretation, *Nursing Diagnosis* 3:123, July/Sept, 1992.
7. Visiting Nurse Association of Omaha. Omaha, Nebr, 1989.
8. Carpenito L: *Nursing diagnosis: application to clinical practice,* ed 2, Philadelphia, 1987, JB Lippincott.
9. Gordon M: *Manual of nursing diagnosis, 1993–1994,* ed 6, St. Louis, 1993, Mosby.
10. Carroll-Johnson R: *Classification of nursing diagnosis: proceedings of the 9th conference,* Philadelphia, 1991, JB Lippincott.
11. McFarland G, McFarlane E: *Nursing diagnosis and intervention,* ed 2, St. Louis, 1993, Mosby.
12. McCourt A: *Syndromes in nursing: a continuing concern; classification of nursing diagnosis: proceedings of the 9th conference,* Philadelphia, 1991, JB Lippincott.
13. Popkess-Vawter S: Nursing diagnosis, wellness nursing diagnoses: to be or not to be? *Nursing Diagnosis* 2:19, Jan/Mar, 1991.
14. Carnevall DL, Thomas MD: *Diagnostic reasoning and treatment decision making in nursing,* Philadelphia, 1993, JB Lippincott.
15. Radwin L: Research on diagnostic reasoning in nursing, *Nursing Diagnosis* 1:70, Apr/June, 1990.
16. Fuller J, Schaller-Ayers J: *Health assessment: a nursing approach,* ed 2, Philadelphia, 1994, JB Lippincott.
17. American Nurses Association Division of Medical Surgical Nursing Practice: *Standards of nursing practice,* Kansas City, Mo, 1974, American Nurses Association.
18. American Nurses Association: *Standards of clinical nursing practice,* Kansas City, Mo, 1991, American Nurses Association.
19. Alfaro-LeFevre R: *Applying nursing process: a step-by-step guide,* ed 3, Philadelphia, 1994, JB Lippincott.
20. Lewis S, Collier I, Heitkemper M: *Medical-surgical nursing: assessment and management of clinical problems,* ed 4, St. Louis, 1996, Mosby.
21. Winningham ML and others: Fatigue and the cancer experience, *Oncology Nursing Forum* 21:28, 1994.

Index

Notes

Notes

Notes

Notes

Notes

Notes

Notes